What people are saying about

Reiki

With Frans Stiene as the guide, t................................ ght
into the depths of Reiki teachings and practice. G........d in
Japanese history, culture, Buddhism and Shintoism, *Reiki Insights*
explores the roots of the system of Reiki. Frans Stiene's writings
allow the reader to deepen and enrich their practice of the Reiki
Precepts, meditations, hands-on-healing, symbols and mantras, to
cultivate mindfulness, healing, compassion, and love.
Elise Brenner, founder and executive director of Celebration of
Reiki, Inc.

I love this book. Frans Stiene has written another inspirational
book, his depth of knowledge about Reiki and ability to share this
knowledge in words we can understand is a gift to us. *Reiki Insights*
is perfect for anyone wishing to deepen their Reiki Meditation
practice, just pick a chapter, read and meditate.
Helen Galpin, co-founder of the British School of Meditation

In *Reiki Insights*, Frans offers practical advice for the lifelong journey
of your Reiki practice: where "life becomes practice and practice
becomes life." Each mini chapter is concise and precise, offering a
wonderful companion to read in conjunction with your daily Reiki
self-care practice and meditation. This will be a must-read for my
Reiki students, and I look forward to rereading it as I continue to
deepen and expand my own practice and understanding of Reiki.
Deborah Flanagan, author of *Building a Powerful Practice: Successful
Strategies for Your Wellness Business*

This profound and powerful book illuminates our understanding
of the true nature of Reiki. Frans Stiene, one of the world's leading

Reiki Teachers, takes us on a journey to the heart of Reiki and unwraps its power to transform and heal.

Mary Pearson, author, *Meditation: the stress solution*

This book is a treasure box, full of magnificent bright precious stones – insights. You can open the box whenever you like and pick a stone, whichever appeals to you at the moment. Every stone is there to read, to play with and to connect to. In the end they all inspire you to get in touch with your True Nature – to feel the gratitude, the beauty and the love that you really are!

Anya van Til, Reiki Waters, the Netherlands

Reading *The Inner Heart of Reiki* and now *Reiki Insights* is like having Frans Stiene here with me. When I read it... I hear his voice, feel the energy, receive the Reiju. Frans Stiene is an exceptional spiritual practitioner so I invite you to feel the stillness between the words. Receive the deep peace that touches the heart, as we continue our journey of remembering the true self. Gratitude to you, Frans, for sharing your clarity and wisdom.

Maria Kammerer, Reiki Practitioner Teacher and founder of Attune: The Art of Reiki

From a holistic nursing perspective, *Reiki Insights* is an exceptional read for all Reiki practitioners working in the field of healthcare. Each concise chapter is a gentle reminder of how we can embody the precepts in order to live in a compassionate and mindful way. Nurturing compassion within ourselves is the key to avoiding burnout in a healthcare system that is often fraught with stress and worry. Frans Stiene, a phenomenal teacher and author, has once again given us a beautiful gift which lovingly guides us on our path to be true to our way and our being.

Helene Williams, BSN, RN, Reiki Teacher/Hospital & Hospice Practitioner, Founder and President, Lancaster Community Reiki Clinic

No one has gone deeper into the true meaning of Mikao Usui's teachings than Frans Stiene. This book shines a clear light on the meditations and practices within the system of Reiki, making them more accessible to the Western mind. With this fuller understanding, the practices themselves come alive and we can take our healing to the deepest of levels.

Joyce Leonard, founder of Santa Cruz Reiki Works

In his latest book, Frans Stiene, the foremost Reiki teacher in the world, takes us farther than ever before into the system of Reiki and the path to our true self. Frans clearly lays out the work that must be done, and then gives us the tools to do it, taking us from the precepts to deep meditations. This is a must-read for anyone who is wanting to not just do Reiki but to be Reiki. To not just talk about spirituality but live a spiritual life.

Jeff Emerson, founder of True Freedom Recovery Yoga

With *Reiki Insights*, world-renowned Reiki teacher Frans Stiene offers yet another gift to the world... and not just to the world of Reiki. He takes us through a journey that takes us back to the beginning, through the end and the middle, to the insight of who we truly are. For Reiki practitioners and seekers, yes, but also for seekers who are being called back into the heart of the matter, this book will help us to reach and touch into who we really are.

Kathryn Hudson, author of *The Angels Told Me So – a practical guide for Lightworkers*

Reiki Insights is for all seekers.

Frans Stiene, acclaimed Reiki teacher, has published an amazing book, *Reiki Insights*. It is amazing because it is not just a Reiki book. It is a book for all spiritual practitioners, whether Reiki or not. In his clear and compassionate manner, Frans Stiene explains the true meaning of the precepts of Mikao Usui. It is only someone who knows, from his own experience after deep practice, that can do this. We are fortunate indeed to receive Mikao Usui's inner teachings as a Way to spiritual freedom from Frans Stiene.

Harriet Natsuyama, author of *The Path Beyond*, okunomichi.wordpress.com

Most of us have only a superficial understanding of the system of Reiki. In this extraordinary work *Reiki Insights*, Frans Stiene, one of the godfathers of Reiki in the West, reveals the system of Reiki to be not only a method of healing, but nothing less than a pathway to enlightenment. If you have ever wanted to explore the deeper meaning of the system of Reiki, this illuminating treasure is for you!

David Michie, author of *The Dalai Lama's Cat* Series

Reiki
Insights

Reiki
Insights

Frans Stiene

AYNI
BOOKS

Winchester, UK
Washington, USA

First published by Ayni Books, 2018
Ayni Books is an imprint of John Hunt Publishing Ltd., No. 3 East Street, Alresford
Hampshire SO24 9EE, UK
office1@jhpbooks.net
www.johnhuntpublishing.com
www.ayni-books.com

For distributor details and how to order please visit the 'Ordering' section on our website.

Text copyright: Frans Stiene 2017

ISBN: 978 1 78535 735 0
978 1 78535 736 7 (ebook)
Library of Congress Control Number: 2017939490

A CIP catalogue record for this book is available from the British Library.

Design: Stuart Davies

Printed and bound by CPI Group (UK) Ltd, Croydon, CR0 4YY, UK

We operate a distinctive and ethical publishing philosophy in
all areas of our business, from our global network of authors to
production and worldwide distribution.

Contents

For my daughter Bella

Foreword

The Japanese character for mankind is 人, you will notice that the representation looks very much like hands praying. Our need as human beings to be spiritually connected is a fundamental element that forms a foundation for a good, happy, and healthy life. We form that character 人 whenever we look into ourselves and pray for our inner goodness to surface. I have known Frans for many years now, and we share our beliefs and thoughts extensively. We both feel that spiritual awareness transcends ideology, and dogma. Compassion and tolerance are not catch words for the ecclesiastic, but rather words we should all strive to live by. In this new book *Reiki Insights*, Frans clearly demonstrates that the understanding of the system of Reiki as a practice begins with clasping your hands in prayer, and letting your inner goodness benefit others.

Rev. Reyn Yorio Tsuru Director of Shingon Shu Hawaii

Preface

Many things have changed since I started to walk the path of the system of Reiki. Change is important as it is how we grow as practitioners and teachers. If we stay still and do not change, we might as well stop the practice altogether. If we do not move from the same spot on our path, maybe because the scenery there is familiar and comfortable to us, then we never can be inspired by the beautiful view we might see just by changing our position. In fact the whole system of Reiki is about facilitating change within oneself.

In 2016 I spent three weeks deep in the mountains of Japan with my own teachers, Shugendo priests who are helping me to gain a deeper understanding of Mikao Usui's teachings through Japanese esoteric teachings. These three weeks were challenging as I confronted my mind, body, and energy, and this brought about many changes within me and the way I see and teach the system of Reiki. Out of these changes grew the writings for my new book *Reiki Insights*, a follow on from *The Inner Heart of Reiki: Rediscovering Your True Self*.

I structured *Reiki Insights* into small chapters so that you can just pick it up, choose a chapter and read it. After you read the chapter, sit down and meditate upon the words. Let them sink deep into your mind, body, and energy, so that you can feel what is in between the sentences. By reading and experiencing *Reiki Insights* in this way, I hope that it might lay a foundation for inner change, change from not knowing your true self to knowing your true self.

My teachers facilitated this change within me and I would like to thank them for guiding me on this path and for helping me to see and teach the system of Reiki from a new place of insight. Thank you, Rev. Takeda Hakusai, Rev. Reyn Yorio Tsuru, and Rev. Kûban Jakkôin. Thank you, Carol Ryan, for editing my work.

Hiromi Hayashi, you have been a great help with the kanji and Japanese translations. I also want to thank all my spiritual friends; without your support this book would never have been written. And thank you to my daughter Bella who is such a bright light, in my life and in the world.

Part 1

The Precepts

Chapter 1

Precepts are Instructions

At the heart of the system of Reiki are the precepts:

> Do not be angry
> Do not worry
> Be grateful
> Practice this diligently
> Show compassion to yourself and others

There are many layers within the precepts and one of these layers is instruction, as the word precept also means instruction. Not only are they instructing us to not be angry and worried, but as the heart of the system of Reiki, the precepts also instruct us how to utilize all other practices within this system.

These other practices are meditation techniques, hands-on healing, symbols and mantras, and the reiju/initiation/attunement.

Let's take a closer look at these instructions and how they relate to some of the practices.

Say we are doing hands-on healing on someone and afterwards they say, "I did not like this session." Often we might get angry or worried, but the precepts instruct us just to let it be.

We often use the word "giving" when we perform hands-on healing on others, or even in connection to the reiju/initiation/attunement. But if we follow the instruction of compassion, then there is nothing to give. Within real compassion there is no giver, gift, and receiver – just being. We also can see this in the kanji of Reiju. Ju 授 means both to give and receive at the same time. Spiritual giving is letting go of the "I" who is giving in the first place. This kind of giving is a natural giving, so natural that we do not even have to call it giving. It is being as natural as the sun; the sun just shines and is not thinking, "I am giving this light to the birds, the people," and so on. It is just shining naturally. So we are not "giving" so much as we are "being" Reiki.

The precepts also are instructing us that we need to practice diligently. Thus we need to practice daily the meditation techniques, practice daily meditations on the symbols and mantras, practice daily hands-on healing on ourselves, practice all aspects of the system of Reiki to deepen our experiences with it.

Being grateful means that we need to be grateful for all of the experiences we have during the practices, no matter if we label them good or bad.

Following these instructions therefore helps us to become more compassionate during our practice, teachings, and daily life.

Chapter 2

The Precepts are for Healing Yourself

Within the Reiki community, we often see just hands-on healing as a means for healing ourselves. But in reality it is not just hands-on healing; the whole system of Reiki consists of tools for healing ourselves.

Healing ourselves means to make whole, and this doesn't always mean fixing a physical issue. Wholeness is a state of mind: a mind in which we feel happy, content, at peace, and full of compassion and insights.

For example, let's look at the Reiki precepts:

Do not anger
Do not worry
Be grateful
Be true to your way and your being
Show compassion to yourself and others

We can just say the precepts three times once a day, which is wonderful. Or we can sit down in meditation and meditate upon the precepts. By meditating on the precepts we start to gain a direct insight into why we get angry, why we get worried, why we do not feel grateful even if we have so many things to appreciate in our lives, why we find it hard to be true to our way and our being, and why we find it difficult to be compassionate to ourselves and others.

But sitting down in meditation takes up more time than just saying the precepts three times, and this is why it is not often taught in a class as a form of healing ourselves.

However, as the precepts are the foundation of the system of Reiki, meditating on the precepts is a very important element of Mikao Usui's teachings as a means for healing ourselves.

What starts to happen when we gain a direct insight into our anger and worry? We start to see why we get angry and worried in the first place. And by seeing this we can take action to soften our anger and worry. If we do not see that we get angry or worried, if we are blind to our own anger and worry, then we cannot do anything about it. Thus a direct insight into our anger and worry helps us to soften the grip on our anger and worry. Instead of clinging tightly to it, we can allow ourselves to feel the anger or worry; we can acknowledge it, and then let it go.

By softening our grip on anger and worry, we start to feel more grateful. And this will move into being more true to our way and our being. By taking that a step further, now we also will become more compassionate to ourselves and others.

Thus we can see that meditating on the precepts is a method for healing ourselves. This in turn will help us to create a more compassionate mind/heart, therefore allowing us to be more compassionate to the world around us. The precepts are directly about healing ourselves, which indirectly has a healing effect on the world around us.

If we look at each practice within Mikao Usui's teachings in this way, we can start to see that meditating on the symbols and mantras is about healing ourselves, that practicing the meditation practices like jōshin kokyū hō is about healing ourselves, that the reiju/ initiation/attunement is about healing ourselves, and that hands-on healing on ourselves and others is about healing ourselves. But remember, healing ourselves is not just physical healing. Real healing – wholeness – is a state of mind/heart in which we have found inner peace, a state of mind/heart filled with compassion and insight.

Chapter 3

On the Wall or In Your Heart?

The precepts are the most important element within the system of Reiki; they are the foundation of the system. Without understanding the foundation, the whole system will crumble like a house without a good solid base.

Some people just stick the precepts on the wall, may recite them a few times a day and that is about it. Some teachers even insist that you must always perform the reiju/initiation/attunement in front of the precepts as they hang on the wall. But merely hanging the precepts on the wall doesn't bring them into your heart.

The real reason the precepts are there is for us to learn to embody them in our hearts. We can only do this by embodying all of the other elements within the system of Reiki. How do we embody them? We do this by meditating upon them. Simply repeating them three times is not enough; we must contemplate what they mean and what their inner secret is. This is not always that easy.

So Mikao Usui also added different tools within his teachings to help us to bring the precepts in our hearts. These tools are meditations: meditating on the mantras and the symbols, meditating with the hand positions, being in a meditative state of mind while performing and receiving the reiju/initiation/attunement, and meditating with techniques like hatsurei hō and jōshin kokyū hō.

If we get too attached to the idea of needing the precepts on the wall to recite, or to see when we do a reiju/initiation/attunement, then we cannot take the wisdom of the precepts out into the big, wide world. When we go out, we are not always carrying the precepts with us on a piece of paper in our pocket. But more importantly, when we carry the precepts in our hearts, we are always ready to be Reiki with others. And to perform reijus/spiritual blessings, we need to embody the precepts in our hearts.

The real secret of the system of Reiki is therefore meditation. And it is by practicing these meditation techniques that we start to bring the precepts from the wall into our hearts, where they really belong.

Chapter 4

Chanting or Reciting the Precepts

One day a student asked me what would be more beneficial, chanting the precepts or reciting them? A complete version follows in English and Japanese, with the words that came before and after the precepts themselves:

The secret method to invite blessings
The spiritual medicine of 10,000 illnesses
Today only
Do not anger
Do not worry
Be grateful
Practice diligently
Show compassion to yourself and others

Perform gassho morning and evening
Bear deeply in your mind/heart
Chant with your mouth
Reform mind/heart and body

Shou fuku no hi hou
Man byoo no rei yaku
Kyo dakewa
Ikaru na
Shinpai Suna
Kansha Shite
Gyō o hageme
Hito ni shinsetsu ni
Asayuu gassho shite
Kokoro ni nenji

Kuchi ni tonae yo
Shinshin kaizen

We often are told to recite the precepts three times, either in Japanese or in our own language. But we all know that just by reciting the precepts three times we will not really embody them. If it were that simple, then by now the whole world would have no more anger and worry, and always would be filled with gratitude and compassion. We would just ask everybody to recite the precepts three times and presto! The world becomes a better place. But as we all know, it is not that simple.

Don't get me wrong; reciting is great. But to recite is to speak from memory, so this can become merely an intellectual experience. Reciting mainly comes from our throat and from our intellectual mind; in the background, our memory/mind tells us "this is the first precept, which is followed by the second precept" and so on. Often this means that reciting only triggers some energy within our heads.

However, Mikao Usui suggested within the precepts themselves that we bear them deeply in our mind/heart. This is done through chanting them. As the precepts say, "Every morning and evening, join your hands in prayer (gassho). Bear deeply in your mind/heart and chant these words with your mouth."

To chant the precepts is something very different from simple recitation. In this case the precepts are seen as a mantra. The word mantra means "protection for the mind."

It protects the mind from not straying into the past, present, and future. This helps keep the mind from getting angry or worried and helps us become more compassionate.

Within Shoden Reiki Level I we learn the meditation jōshin kokyū hō in which we breathe deeply into the hara/tanden. This practice, called okinagaho in Japanese, triggers deep, long breathing and helps to increase power in the physical body. This power can then be used, for example, to help us not get angry or worried and to be compassionate to ourselves and others.

The deep long breathing also ensures that when we use the precepts as a mantra, the sound emanates from the center of our being, from the hara/tanden. Thus the energy being released through chanting can travel throughout our whole being, not just within our head. This way we start to bear the precepts deeply in our mind/heart, and not just in our memory.

But even if we chant the mantra just three times like this, that doesn't make much change either. Therefore to really bear the precepts in our mind/heart we need to chant them for a prolonged period of time, maybe 20 minutes for example. This will help to rest our mind on our hara/tanden because of the deep long breathing, which in turn helps us to become more grounded and centered. This in turn helps us to become less angry and worried. You see all the practices within the system of Reiki are interrelated.

Of course we can say it is semantics, recite vs. chant, but that depends on how we recite. If we recite with the deep long breathing pattern from our hara/tanden, then reciting becomes mantra.

So which is better, chanting or reciting? Both are good as long as we recite or chant for a prolonged period of time and the sounds come from our hara/tanden, our center. This will help us to embody the precepts more and more so that we can become the precepts.

When an experienced practitioner talks, his words have a blessed energy. He may be talking about the same thing the scholars are, but the way he expresses himself touches your heart. The talk of those without experience is like the empty wind whistling about your ears.

– Lama Thubten Yeshe, *When the Chocolate Runs Out*

So, as we deepen our practice, we expand our experience. As we expand our experience, our words and the way we express them takes on more and more of this blessed energy, as Lama Thubten Yeshe says. So whether reciting or chanting, let's go deeper in our practice with the precepts. In doing this, our words will touch not only our own heart, but others' hearts as well.

Chapter 5

Spiritual Medicine

Within the precepts we see the phrase "spiritual medicine." But what does spiritual medicine stand for?

> The secret of inviting happiness through many blessings
> The spiritual medicine for all illness
>
> For today only:
> Do not anger
> Do not worry
> Be grateful
> Practice diligently
> Be compassionate to yourself and others

One day I was reading though a wonderful book, *Immortal Sisters: Secrets of Taoist Women*, translated and edited by Thomas Cleary. In it, I came across this interesting quote:

> Attentively guard the spiritual medicine, with every breath return to the beginning of the creative.

It goes on to say, "The spiritual medicine is subtle being, and subtle being means true breathing. So attentively guarding the spiritual medicine means keeping the attention on the breathing."

Within this quote they say that the spiritual medicine is subtle being. For me this subtle being is our true self, our essence. But the quote goes even further; to be able to stay in this state of mind of true self/subtle being, we need to keep our attention on the breathing. This is why Mikao Usui not only put meditation practices like jōshin kokyū hō and hatsurei hō within his system, but also included mantras in his teachings. When we chant a mantra, we perform deep breathing. Our attention is not just on the sound, but also on the deep breathing which is essential to the mantra.

But why is placing our attention on our breathing so important to guard our spiritual medicine, our true self? When we place our attention on our breathing, we are mindful. We do not stray into the past, present, and future. To guard our spiritual medicine, our true self, we need to be mindful not to cover it up with worry, fear, and anger. And this we do through keeping our attention on our breathing. We get angry or worried because we stray into the past, present, and future. This is really what the precepts are pointing out.

Imagine getting worried; what is our mind doing? It is going into the past or future. But if we are putting our attention on our breathing, it stays in the moment and therefore we are not getting worried.

If we get angry, but then we start to focus on our breathing, what happens? We have created a pause, some patience. By placing our attention on our breathing rather than following our anger, this pause will help us to let go of our anger.

This is why all the breathing practices within the system of Reiki are so important: they all are tied in with the precepts.

To sum it all up, the real spiritual medicine is our true self, and the precepts are pointers. And to help ourselves to embody the precepts, we place our attention on our breathing. This is guarding our spiritual medicine, minding our true self.

Chapter 6

Do Not Bear Anger for Anger is an Illusion

Within the system of Reiki, the first precept says this: Do not anger.

However, it is said that Mikao Usui also was teaching a more elaborate precept about anger to some of his Buddhist students. That precept goes like this: Do not bear anger for anger is an illusion.

It is not hard to get an intellectual grasp of what the word "bear" means in this precept. "Do not bear anger" really means do not carry it around with you. Just observe it arising; don't bear it, and it will dissolve all by itself.

However, "anger is an illusion" is much harder to grasp.

In 2016 I met up with Orgyen Chowang in California who wrote a wonderful book called *Our Pristine Mind: A Practical Guide to Unconditional Happiness*.

In his book he writes very clearly about what illusion means and how this relates to anger. Here is a quote from his book:

Illusoriness is sometimes misunderstood to mean that there is nothing there. If nothing appeared, however, we would not refer to it as an illusion because there would be no object to be an illusion. The point of illusoriness is that there seems to be something there, but doesn't really exist as we think it does. Something appears, and in ordinary mind we are convinced something is real, but what we think it is in actuality does not exist in the way it appears.

"Anger is an illusion" therefore doesn't mean that anger is not there. It is there but it does not exist in the way it appears; it does not exist in the way we may think it does.

Chowang also states: "... if we pay attention to our anger and other negative emotions, they grow more powerful; if we do not pay attention to them, they disappear. "This quote really points to the word "bear." If we pay no attention to our anger it will dissolve. Or in other words, if we do not bear our anger it will dissolve.

Orgyen Chowang continues with, "When we do this, the angry energy fades away into nothingness because it was an illusion. Anger is an illusory appearance like the rainbow and the clouds. Circumstances and our perception make that anger appear. When we look closely at that anger, when we focus on the energy of anger and look directly at it, our perception shifts; we see there is nothing really there that we can identify as 'anger.'"

This is why it is so important to not just recite the precepts mindlessly, but to really investigate what they mean and how they relate to our own way of living. We have to look really closely at our anger so that, as Chowang suggests above, our perception of the anger shifts. We can do this through the meditation practices taught within the system of Reiki and by meditating on the precepts.

Orgyen Chowang emphasizes this point by saying: "In the same way, when we hear about illusoriness, our habit of assuming that things really are as they appear is so strong that it is hard to convince us that mental events are illusions. This is why illusoriness is very difficult for us to really understand. Even when we gain some intellectual understanding of it, the real meaning of illusoriness is something that has to be experienced through familiarity with meditation. "This is why the system of Reiki is a lifelong practice. And this is why it is so important to apply the meditation practices which Mikao Usui put into his system, so that we can have the direct experience of why anger is an illusion.

He explains it even further: "If thoughts and emotions like anger, desire, jealousy, and all other mental events are illusions, why do they have such power? It is because we do not realize that they are illusions." Again, this is why we have to apply the meditation practices within the system of Reiki so that we can realize that our emotions are illusions. Not just anger but worry, jealousy, and "other mental events."

Orgyen Chowang continues, "Sometimes people think we are denying or dismissing their emotional experiences if we say that mental events are illusions. They can become defensive. But identifying mental events as illusory is not intended to discount them. Of course, they do seem real, powerful, and able to affect our life. The point is that they are not the way they seem, and they do not have to have the powerful grip over us that we give them. That is why it is so transformative to understand their illusory nature." Mikao Usui was pointing out the same, that it is healing to understand the illusory nature of anger.

Thoughts come and go all throughout our lives. But if we focus on them and label, judge or distinguish, then we bear them in our mind and we give them power, power to become anger or worry. But before the moment we label, judge, or distinguish our thoughts, they are neither positive nor negative; they are just energy.

As Orgyen Chowang points out, "Mental events do not have any inherent power apart from what we bestow on them with our attention. We perceive them as real, and that perception makes them powerful. Even if something is not real, if we think it is real, then it becomes powerful to us." As we can see, the precepts hold a lot of important teachings to rediscover and embody through our daily meditation practices as Mikao Usui taught. Because it is through the direct experience of embodying the precepts that real healing starts to take place. And realizing that anger is an illusion, as in the first precept, is a first step on the path to healing.

Chapter 7

Gyō o Hageme – Work Hard?

Do not anger
Do not worry
Be grateful
Be true to your true self
Show compassion to yourself and others

Within the system of Reiki we have the five precepts. In Japanese, the fourth precept is gyō o hageme.

Most of the time gyō o hageme is translated as work hard or work diligently.

But gyō o hageme can mean so much more than work hard! Let's take a closer look.

Gyō is often translated as work or practice; however, it also means karma, pure experience, action, and function.

Directly translated, hageme means hard or diligently, but it also can mean to strive, inspire, encourage, or to wholeheartedly devote oneself to a cause.

The pure experience of gyō is the natural expression of our inner state of mind. It is a direct experience of our true self; hence, it is pure without any ego. This pure experience starts to happen when we let go of our anger and worry and when we are being grateful to all that is. It is the direct pure experience which comes from practicing the meditation practices that Mikao Usui put in his teachings.

Now let's look at different translations of gyō o hageme:

- Devote oneself wholeheartedly to your pure experience. Or in other words, be true to your true self.
- Strive to express yourself through your pure experience.
- Inspire through your pure experience.

When we inspire others through our pure experience, then this is really compassion. And we can only inspire others when we have let go of our anger and worry and when we are grateful for all that happens on our path.

Thus when looking at gyō o hageme, we can find so much more than work hard. In fact if we look at the deeper meaning of gyō o hageme, we start to see that Mikao Usui's teachings are a real spiritual practice. In this practice, we are striving to lay bare our pure experience so that we can inspire others to do the same.

> For mountain ascetics, gyō is to live according to the spirit of that precept.
> – Ryōjun Shionuma

So as we practice the system of Reiki, let us strive not only "to live according to the spirit of that precept" – gyō o hageme – but also to live according to the spirit of each one of the precepts.

Chapter 8

Be Kind to Yourself and Others

Within the system of Reiki we have the precepts and one precept is this:

hito ni shinsetsu ni
人 に 親切 に
Be kind to people

This precept is often translated as "Be kind to others."

The kanji of 人 hito means people, human beings and person. The kanji hito does not mean others! However, in our modern society we often look outside of ourselves, always projecting externally. And therefore hito has been mistranslated as others.

But we cannot separate ourselves from people; we cannot separate ourselves from human beings, as we are people and human beings as well. Thus the real meaning for "hito ni shinsetsu ni" is "be kind to yourself and others." In "other" words – we are others and others are us. So whatever translation is used, this precept points to kindness to all.

> I and others have the same root. All beings and myself are in unity.
> – Taisen Deshimaru, *Mushotoku Mind: The Heart of the Heart Sutra*

I always say, "I cannot give you tea if I do not have tea." I cannot be kind to others if I am not kind to myself; both have to go hand in hand.

According to the *Dictionary of Buddhism*, hito also means "self" and "ego."

Thus we also can translate the phrase in this way: Be kind to your self – your ego. This really means let go of the self – let go of the ego, as this is the deepest form of kindness you can show yourself.

And what is the deepest form of kindness you can show others? Show them how to let go of their ego!

When we have let go of our ego, we realize that one and others are of the same root and cannot be separated. One and others are in unity. So when we go inside to find and cultivate kindness in ourselves and for ourselves, when we step away from our ego and external view of "others," we can find and cultivate kindness in all.

Chapter 9

Spiritual Blessings

Within Mikao Usui's teachings we come across this sentence: "The esoteric teachings to invite blessings," which is seen in the prelude of the precepts. A translation of the full text included with the precepts follows:

The esoteric teachings to invite blessings
The spiritual medicine of having strayed from universal truth

Today only
Do not anger
Do not worry
Be grateful
Be true to your way and your true self
Show compassion to yourself and others
Perform gassho in the morning and evening
Embody this in your mind/heart
Chant with your mouth
Improve your mind/heart and body

Usui's teachings to remember one's true self
The founder, Mikao Usui

Many practitioners and teachers believe that the blessings Mikao Usui is talking about within this statement refer to the reiju/initiation/attunement. But this is not the case. If we look deeply into the whole statement, we do not come across the concept of reiju/initiation/attunement at all. Rather, we come across a specific state of mind, a state of mind of no anger, no worry, of being grateful, of being true to our way and our true self, and of being compassionate to ourselves and others.

The real blessing Mikao Usui is talking about is one of embodying this state of mind in our mind/heart all day long; that is the blessing.

Think about it.

Wouldn't it be a blessing if we do not have to get angry anymore and if we do not have to deal with angry people?

Wouldn't it be a blessing if we don't have to worry and fear anymore and if we don't have to deal with worried and fearful people?

Wouldn't it be a blessing if we can be grateful for everything which comes our way no matter what?

Wouldn't it be a blessing if we can live a life of being true to our way and our true self and not to another person's way?

Wouldn't it be a blessing if we can be compassionate all the time to ourselves and others and that other people are compassionate to us and themselves?

These kinds of blessings are also self-induced, which means we feel strong and empowered from within. They come from our own personal practice when we meditate on the precepts, meditate during hands-on healing, meditate on the symbols and mantras, practice the meditation practices like jōshin kokyū hō, and be meditative when we practice reiju/initiation/attunement.

If we think that the blessing Mikao Usui is talking about is the reiju/initiation/attunement itself, then this means that we always have to rely on an external source, the teacher who performs the reiju/initiation/attunement. This creates a state of dependency and is not empowering at all. Because we cannot be with the teacher 24/7, the teacher is there to help us to empower ourselves so that we can feel these internal blessings – a state of mind of no anger, no worry, gratitude, being true to our way and our true self, and being compassionate – all day and night long. We can feel these blessings on our own without depending on the teacher to bestow or ignite them.

Therefore delve deep into the heart of the system of Reiki and feel the blessings of embodying the precepts in your daily life; feel these blessings raining down on you all the time.

Chapter 10

Reiki and Acceptance

When we delve deep into the system of Reiki, we rediscover acceptance.

Acceptance is a very important element in healing ourselves and helping other people to heal themselves. Without acceptance, we start to fight and struggle with ourselves and others.

Let's take a look at the precepts:

Do not anger
Do not worry
Be grateful
Be true to your way and your true self
Show compassion to yourself and others

When we perform hands-on treatments with someone else, we have to do this from a place of acceptance. If we feel the need to protect ourselves during a session, then there is no acceptance. Protecting ourselves comes from a place of fear and worry, a place where we do not accept our clients for who they are. Thus the more we let go of our worry and fear, the more we start to accept others. The more we accept others, the more freely our energy flows and the more open spaciousness we can offer our clients to start healing themselves.

But of course this also reflects back to ourselves. Often we do not accept ourselves for who we are and where we are at in our personal practice and life. If we do not accept ourselves, if we are always fighting with aspects of ourselves, this in turn creates anger, worry, and fear.

Accepting ourselves is like placing ourselves and our issues in an open hand, the open hand of acceptance. For example, when we have a disease, we often fight with it and this creates worry, fear, and anger. This kind of fighting is a struggle between us and the disease. And in this fight we are holding our issue in a tight fist, the closed fist of struggling. When our fist is closed, our mind is closed and thus our energy is not flowing freely. But when we open the hand of acceptance, our mind also becomes more open and our energy starts to flow more freely. This free-flowing energy therefore will create a better environment for healing to take place.

Accepting is therefore intertwined with being grateful. Being grateful means accepting everything that comes our way no matter what. This kind of gratefulness comes from our open expanded compassionate state of mind, which includes everybody and everything. Or in other words, this kind of acceptance is compassion.

Being compassionate to ourselves and others is all about acceptance: accepting ourselves with all our "good" and "bad" issues and accepting others with all their "good" and "bad" issues. Good and bad are between "" marks to remind us that when we go deeper into rediscovering our true self we start to see that we are all a great bright light, no matter what our outer layers are. And when we start to see this great bright light in ourselves and others, then there is no more division and pure acceptance is born.

Chapter 11

How to Boost Your Energy with the Precepts

The precepts are the foundation of the system of Reiki.

Do not anger
Do not worry
Be grateful
Be true to your way and your being
Show compassion to yourself and others

There are many teachings to be discovered within the precepts, and one of these is energy – ki. The precepts point towards preserving our energy.

Do you get tired quickly or, more to the point, do you feel depleted after you get angry or feel worried? Do you feel drained after you are boasting, lying, or being unkind?

Most of us do. But why is this? When we get angry or worried we are expending our energy, draining it. This also happens when we are boasting about ourselves, lying about things, or when we are unkind to ourselves and others. If we spend all our energy with these issues, then we have little left to nourish our own being, let alone to help others.

Let's look at an example. Where is our mind when we are worried? It is in the past or the future because that is what we worry about. If our mind is in the past or the future, where is our energy? Our energy is also in the past or the future, because energy follows our mind. If our energy is in the past and the future, then we have no energy to sustain ourselves at this moment. If we have no energy to sustain ourselves, then quickly we become tired, stressed, and depleted.

The precepts therefore point towards nourishing and cultivating our own inner energy so that we can live a healthier and happier life. If we do not deplete our own inner energy, we start to feel stronger, happier, healthier, and less tired.

This is also why we need to practice the system of Reiki when we are still healthy. If we wait until we get sick or depressed, our energy is already weakening; thus we do not have much energy to bring us back to a healthier state. But if we have a strong internal energy before we get sick or depressed, we can fall back on the surplus to help us heal more quickly.

Now we also can see why Mikao Usui taught meditation practices like the jōshin kokyū hō breathing method: to be in a state of mind of concentration. If we are concentrating on our breath, we will get less angry and worried and thus we are conserving our energy. The precepts and all the meditation practices within the system of Reiki are there to help us sustain our own inner energy for our own well-being. And with continued practice, we can continue to sustain and to boost our energy throughout our lives.

Chapter 12

Reiki On – Reiki Off

One day I heard someone say that when we do hands-on healing on ourselves, we switch "Reiki on" and that when we do not place our hands on or slightly off our body, we switch "Reiki off."

For me Reiki means our true self; we do not want to switch that off. In fact, we want to keep it on day and night. Our true self is like a great bright light, so why would we switch it off or cover it up? Let it shine day and night because it is in this brightness that healing takes place – healing for ourselves and for everybody and everything else.

Reiki can be directly translated as spiritual energy. Wouldn't it be great if we could remember this spiritual energy 24 hours a day and not just switch it on when we do hands-on healing?

For me Reiki is the precepts, because we can only really embody the precepts when we lay bare our spiritual energy, our true self, our Reiki, in its fullest.

> The precepts are...
> Do not anger
> Do not worry
> Be grateful
> Be true to your way and your true self
> Show compassion to yourself and others

So when we say, "Reiki on," then we are kind of saying, "Switch the precepts on." And when we say, "Reiki off," we are kind of saying that we are switching the precepts off. Reiki, spiritual energy, our true self cannot be distinguished from the precepts; they are one and the same. Wouldn't it be great to stay in that state of mind/heart of the precepts 24 hours a day?! What a change this would make in our daily life and in our world.

Switching Reiki on and off also comes from a very dualistic viewpoint. However, when we go deeper into our own personal practice within the system of Reiki, we start to realize that there is no Reiki on and off; there is just being Reiki 24 hours a day.

So again, for me Reiki means our true self, like our great bright light. So why would we switch it off or cover it up? It is in this brightness that healing takes place. So let your light shine bright both day and night!

Chapter 13

The 3 Actions of the Reiki Precepts

Do not anger
Do not worry
Be grateful
Practice diligently
Show compassion to yourself and others

Within Japanese Buddhism there are three main precepts, which encompass all other precepts that you can find within Japanese Buddhism. We can see that Mikao Usui based his five precepts on these three main precepts.

Let's investigate how the precepts within the system of Reiki fall underneath these three main Japanese Buddhist precepts.

1 – sho ritsu kai – cease to do bad actions

Within Usui's precepts, the "bad actions" we are to cease are being angry and worried. It is simple yet so hard to do as we are so caught up in all our attachments that we can find it very difficult to cease our anger and worry.

2 – sho jen bo kai – do good actions

Usui's precepts show us four steps related to doing good actions. The first is the good actions we do so that others do not get angry and worried. We often may think that the precepts only point to ourselves not getting angry and worried, but in performing these healthy actions, we help others to not get angry and worried themselves. The second step is being grateful in our lives. In the good action of being grateful, we cease to do bad actions; gratefulness helps us to accept things as they are and to stop getting angry and worried about what has been or what may be. This of course only can happen when we practice diligently, which is the third step. The fourth step is the action of being compassionate to ourselves.

But, you may ask, what about being compassionate to others? This falls under the third main precept...

3 – sho shu jo kai – the action of helping others

Helping others is by being compassionate to others. But what does being compassionate to others really mean, what does helping others really mean? We can say it means to help the old lady with her shopping bag, or offering a hands-on healing session to someone. But that is the basic level of being compassionate. A deeper level of being compassionate is the action of helping others to remember their own true self. If we help others to remember their own true self, they will cease to do bad actions, will perform good actions, and will help others to remember their true self. Now the ripple effect of the three actions will spread around the world.

However, helping others, within both the Reiki precepts and the Buddhist precepts, comes last because if we help others and we still have lot of anger and worry within ourselves, then we are not really helping others at all.

Being a Buddhist practitioner himself, it is not surprising that Mikao Usui based his precepts around all of this. Just as each precept within each system is deeply interrelated to the others, the three precepts and the five precepts also are interrelated. Simple yet complex. Clear yet multilayered.

As you can see, there are many things to discover within Mikao Usui's teachings. And by following these three actions – cease to do bad; do good; help others – we start to embody the system of Reiki more and more in our daily lives. This in turn will create a more compassionate world.

Chapter 14

Bodhichitta and the System of Reiki

Bodhichitta is the intent or aspiration to gain enlightenment to benefit all sentient beings. Bodhichitta is a Sanskrit word. Bodhi means wisdom, and Chitta means mind/heart; thus it stands for a mind/heart full of wisdom. This wisdom is that we want to rediscover our true self/Reiki so that we can help others to rediscover their true self/Reiki.

Mikao Usui showed this to us as well in his precepts! Yes indeed, all we have to do is look deeply within the precepts, and we can find it there. The precept "show compassion to yourself and others" points towards bodhichitta. What does "show compassion to yourself and others" mean on the deepest level? Exactly this: that we gain enlightenment (rediscovery of our true self/Reiki) by showing compassion to ourselves, and this will benefit all sentient beings, by showing compassion to others.

Some might say that Bodhichitta is a Buddhist concept. But in reality it is a universal concept; Bodhichitta is just the Buddhist name. Mikao Usui called it, "show compassion to yourself and others," while other traditions might call it Universal Love.

The Secret of Inviting Happiness through Many Blessings
The Spiritual Medicine for All Illness

For today only:
Do not anger
Do not worry
Be grateful

Be true to your way and your being
Be compassionate to yourself and others

A mind/heart full of wisdom and compassion (this is our true self/ Reiki) is the real spiritual medicine Mikao Usui pointed out in his precepts, for rediscovering this will bring great inner happiness. And the blessing is that as we aspire to rediscover our true self/ Reiki, we can help others too, along the way.

Chapter 15

The Reiki Precepts and the Six Paramitas

When I have shown the Reiki precepts to Japanese Buddhist teachers (for example Shugendo, Shingon, and Tendai priests), they point out that the precepts are linked to the six paramitas. Takeda Ajari, an esteemed Shingon priest, feels that Mikao Usui created the Reiki precepts to allow his students to have a direct experience of the six paramitas without actually pointing the six paramitas out to them. This might have been done because in Mikao Usui's time the Meiji Emperor decided to separate the religions of Shinto and Buddhism in Japan. State Shinto was introduced and was promoted in the name of national unity and patriotic duty. Therefore, Mikao Usui might have created a simple form of the six paramitas which was more accessible to people who had to practice State Shinto.

The Reiki precepts are listed here in Japanese:

Kyo dake wa
Ikaru-na
Shinpai suna
Kansha shite
Gyō o hage me
Hito ni shin-setsu ni

This can be translated in different ways depending not only on how the kanji is read, but also on the spiritual state of mind of the translator. I personally like this translation of the precepts:

For today only
Do not anger
Do not worry

Be grateful
Practice diligently
Show compassion to yourself and others

The six paramitas are listed here:

Generosity
Morality
Patience
Persistence
Concentration
Wisdom

Let's have a look and see how the Reiki precepts and the six paramitas intertwine with each other.

Generosity means giving and sharing. In Japanese Buddhism, there are different elements of giving. One is the gift of material things, but a much more generous gift is the gift of no more fear. The gift of no more fear is that as people we do not become angry, so we do not instill fear in others. Fear is also interlinked with worry; when we do not worry, we become calmer and therefore can radiate that calmness out to others.

One of the most generous gifts we can give to others is to share the teachings on how to embody the Reiki precepts in their daily lives. If everyone embodied the precepts, the world would be a better place for all of us, people and animals alike. Real giving also needs to come from an egoless state of mind, giving without strings attached. This in essence means that we have a state of mind in which there is no giver, no gift, and no receiver. This can only start to happen when we let go of the ego, the "I." Mikao Usui pointed this out in the precepts as well, because when we let go of the "I," then there is no "I" who gets angry or worried. There is no "I" who gets in the way of being grateful and compassionate. And there is no "I" who gets in the way of not practicing diligently.

Morality means that we have to look at our moral conduct: moral conduct is the embodiment of the precepts. There are three elements of morality. The first is refraining from negative actions, like anger and worry. We often think worry is for ourselves, but it also is about not instilling worry in someone else. The second element is about accumulating positive actions, which links to being grateful. We have to be grateful for all things in life, for it is only through being grateful for both "good" and "bad" that we start to be positive in life. And the third aspect of morality is helping others, which is of course linked in with showing compassion to others. The deepest form of compassion we can show to others is in helping them to rediscover their true self, their essence, because it is only in that state of rediscovery that they can start to really heal themselves.

The paramita of patience is about acceptance. This not only is linked to being grateful but also to anger. When we are patient with someone we will get less angry with them, and also will be less angry within ourselves. Patience therefore is the real antidote to anger.

Persistence is linked to practicing diligently. Without practicing diligently the meditation practices Mikao Usui placed in his teachings, we will not start to embody the precepts in our heart; they will be merely empty words that we repeat. Therefore the deeper aspect of persistence is the willingness to embody the precepts in our life so that we can help others. Persistence is therefore also interlinked with compassion. The deepest level of compassion we can show to ourselves is the willingness to rediscover our true self, our essence, because it is only at this stage that we can help others to find their true self. If we don't know how to find it ourselves, how can we help others to do so?

Concentration is about meditative concentration, so that we do not get angry and worried. We get angry or worried because we are not mindful, not focused. The deepest aim of concentration is rediscovering our true self and it is only from this rediscovery that we can embody the precepts in all we do. This in turn will create a better world, because if we do not get angry and worried, if we are grateful and compassionate, then this state of mind/heart will have a huge healing effect on everything around us.

Wisdom is about the complete embodiment of the precepts.

This wisdom is the foundation for no more anger and no more worry.

This wisdom is the base on which we can rest our gratitude for whatever happens to us.

This wisdom gives us strength and energy to practice diligently.

This wisdom shows us a clear path to being compassionate to ourselves and others.

As you can see, the Reiki precepts are in fact no different than the six paramitas. If we embody the five Reiki precepts, we also are embodying the six paramitas; the two are one and the same.

Part 2

Reiki in Daily Life

Chapter 16

How to Strengthen Your Inner Energy with Reiki

According to the World Health Organization, more than 350 million people around the world suffer from depression. On their website they describe some of the symptoms of depression as reduced energy leading to diminished activities and a loss of enjoyment.

What is the reason we feel a loss of energy and joy in our daily life?

Most of the time it is because of our state of mind. Energy (Japanese – Ki) follows the mind; thus if the mind is all over the place due to fear, worry, and anger, we start to feel depleted of energy. In our modern age we are also so distracted and busy with all sorts of external things: Facebook, iPhones, computers, TV, mortgages, work, worrying about what other people think of what we say and do, you name it. These distractions create a scattered mind and therefore a scattered and depleted internal energy. This in turn makes us feel less energetic, less joyful, less compassionate, and it creates a lack of clarity.

The system of Reiki was created to bring this scattered mind home, back into our own center.

This center is called the hara/tanden and it is located a few fingers' width below your navel. Stand up and place your hand there; look at your hand and discover that this is the center of your body, right in the center between your feet and crown! Think of the many times you have felt "off center" or "out of balance." The practices of Reiki can bring you back to center, back into balance.

One of the most important practices within the system of Reiki is jōshin kokyū hō, which translates as "breathing method to be in a state of mind of concentration." When our minds are in a state of concentration, we are staying in the present moment. We are not caught up with unnecessary worries and fears which deplete our inner energy. When we learn to be present, our minds become calm and thus our energy becomes calm. This kind of concentration is called mindfulness. We are being mindful of not spending our inner energy on anger, worry, fear, boasting, lying, and being unkind. Thus, through concentration/being mindful we are generating more energy!

We all have the ability to generate this energy of mindfulness.
– Thich Nhat Hanh, *You Are Here: Discovering the Magic of the Present Moment*

We can use this energy to heal our own issues like depression, stress, and other health problems.

Imagine your center as a pot filled with energy and joy. If we always keep scattering things out of this pot in all directions, to the past and future, then there will be nothing left in the pot. If we have an empty pot we start to feel that we have less energy to do things; we quickly get tired and angry, and we start to feel stressed and unhappy.

But if we bring our mind back to our inner center, our inner pot, we start to fill it up with fresh clear energy. This energy is full of joy and happiness that we can use for dealing with our issues. And what if we practice this meditation daily? We might even feel that this pot/our center is overflowing with healthy, joyful, clear, strong, mindful energy! It can become so full that it starts to overflow in all directions. We can use this overflowing energy to help others to fill up their depleted pots of energy without depleting our own pot, because our own pot is overflowing! This is just one example of a specific practice taught within the system of Reiki. All the other practices, like the symbols and mantras, the precepts, reiju/initiation, meditation practices, and hands-on healing are tools to help us to create an open compassionate state of mind in which our own inner energy is so overflowing with love, that it spills out into the world.

Chapter 17

Reiki and Mindfulness

When we start to look deeply within the system of Reiki, we begin to see that Mikao Usui really is teaching us about our state of mind and how to work with the mind.

This, of course, makes perfect sense since we all know that energy follows the mind.

- If the mind is distracted, our energy is also distracted.
- If our mind is all over the place, our energy is also all over the place.
- If our energy is all over the place, we do not have any focused energy within to heal ourselves let alone help others to heal themselves.

So how did Mikao Usui show us that the system of Reiki is all about the mind?

Here are 4 examples of how Mikao Usui helps us to understand about the mind by practicing the system of Reiki.

1. The first example is the precepts:

Do not anger
Do not worry
Be grateful
Be true to your way and your being
Be compassionate to yourself and others

The precepts talk about a state of mind: a state of mind of

peacefulness, openness, calmness, and inclusiveness.

The precepts do not talk about the physical aspect of hands-on healing, which really can only take place when the mind is calm. This is why Mikao Usui placed the precepts at the foundation of the system of Reiki.

2. The second example is the meditations taught within the traditional Japanese system of Reiki. With each in breath we focus on the hara/tanden, just below our navel; this helps us to stay focused in the present moment. Each time we become distracted, we bring the mind (and therefore also the energy) back to the hara. It is not unlike tying the mind to one specific point, so that it is unable to roam. By repeating this practice, we train the mind to remain focused and to not become distracted.

3. The third example is the symbols and mantras. Mantra is known as a protection of the mind. By allowing us to focus on one specific word and sound, giving us control over our wandering mind, the mantra therefore is protecting it from straying. Once again, we need to do this practice again and again and again so that we can become used to having a focused mind.

The same can be said of our symbol practice. The symbol is a tool we've been given to support us in focusing, enabling the mind to stay with one focal point.

4. And the fourth example is mindfulness. All of these Reiki practices come under the heading of mindfulness training. To be mindful, we need to ask ourselves this: what do we need to be mindful of?

We need to be mindful of not clinging to issues of the past, future, and present. And the tools within the system of Reiki are helping us to do just that – be mindful.

So stay focused to bring your mind under control so that you have plenty of focused energy to heal yourself and to help others to heal themselves too.

Chapter 18

Energy Follows the Mind

If our mind is all over the place our energy also is all over the place.

As energy follows the mind, it is of utmost importance to make sure that when we practice the system of Reiki, our mind is focused, clear, open, and expanded. A focused, clear, open, expanded mind means that our energy is also focused, clear, open, and expanded.

In many of his teachings, Mikao Usui also pointed out that energy follows the mind.

The precepts are a perfect example of this:

Today only
Do not anger
Do not worry
Be grateful
Be true to your way and your true self
Show compassion to yourself and others

For today really means in the present moment. Keeping our mind in the present moment helps us to let go of a lot of our anger and worry, because often we are angry and worried about something which happened in the past. Being grateful is having an open expanded state of mind so that we can accept things as they are, without judging or getting angry and worried about them. This in turn will create a more compassionate state of mind. We all know that we can kind of feel this in people's energy. If an angry person walks into a room, often we can feel this; it is tangible in their energy. If a happy person walks into the room, often we can feel this as well; their happy energy touches our heart and we start to feel joyful ourselves.

Precepts also mean instructions: by giving us signposts for how to create a calm, grateful, compassionate state of mind, the precepts are instructing us how to perform hands-on healing. This thus means that Mikao Usui was teaching us to let go of all our anger and worry, to be grateful, to be organic – true to our way and our true self – and to be compassionate during a session. He knew that if our mind is not in the right place, our energy also is not in the right place. This in turn means that if our mind is not in the right place, our hands-on healing session also is not in the right place. If our energy is infused with anger and worry, and not infused with gratefulness, being organic, and having compassion, it's almost as if our session is taking place in the room with the angry person we mentioned above, not the happy person.

Another practice which points out that energy follows the mind is hatsurei hō. It is a meditation practice which helps us to become more focused, clear, open, and expanded. Mikao Usui placed this within his system to help us to calm our mind and energy so that when we want to support others in their healing journey, we can do this in a clear, open state of mind and energy.

The symbols are yet another tool to calm our mind and energy. When we get distracted by the past, present, and future, we can focus on the symbols so that our mind gets focused again on what we are doing. This in turn will make our energy more focused. Hon sha ze sho nen is pointing clearly to a clear state of mind: literally hon sha ze sho nen translates as "my true nature is right mindfulness."

Mikao Usui placed all of these pointers within his teachings because he knew that to help others, to be compassionate to others, we need to have the right mindfulness within ourselves – first being compassionate to ourselves – because energy follows the mind.

Chapter 19

Reiki is Meditation

In essence, meditation is not a specific posture or a way of breathing, but it is a state of mind. And meditation practices help us to lay bare this specific state of mind.

Let's first look at how meditation practices are essential to the system of Reiki.

Mikao Usui taught meditation practices which focus on the hara/tanden just below the navel: they are jōshin kokyū hō, seishin toitsu and hatsurei hō. Utilizing breath and visualization, these practices help us to have a direct experience of a meditative state of mind.

In her diary, Mrs. Takata, who brought the system of Reiki to the West, wrote about the importance of meditation practices within the system of Reiki. Here is a diary excerpt from December 10th, 1935:

Meaning of "Reiki" Energy within oneself, when concentrated and applied to patient, will cure all ailments – it is nature's greatest cure, which requires no drugs. It helps in all respects, human and animal life. In order to concentrate, one must purify one's thoughts in words and in thoughts and to meditate to let the "energy" come out from within. It lies in the bottom of the stomach about 2 inches below the navel. Sit in a comfortable position, close your eyes, concentrate on your thoughts and relax…

Here she is clearly pointing out that to let the true "energy" [Reiki] come out from within, we need to meditate.

But jōshin kokyū hō, seishin toitsu and hatsurei hō are not the only practices we can use as meditation. Mikao Usui also taught meditation practices with the symbols and mantras. By resting and concentrating our mind on the symbols, we can reach a state of mind of meditation. By chanting the mantras, which include deep breathing into the hara/tanden, we also purify our thoughts. Through this, we again can reach a state of mind of meditation.

The precepts are also a meditation practice. Writing this at the end of the precepts, Mikao Usui clearly instructed us to meditate:

心 に 念じ
kokoro ni nenji
Mind/heart to pray silently

口 に 　　唱へ よ
kuchi ni tonae yo
mouth at chant do

In other words, he says, "Bear deeply in your mind/heart and chant these words with your mouth."

To chant the precepts with our mouth means that we have to chant them out loud. To do this, we have to breathe deeply into the hara/tanden so that the sound of the chanting can resonate through our whole being. By chanting the precepts, we also concentrate our mind, and the vibration of the chanting will help us to purify our thoughts. All of this shows that chanting the precepts is a meditation practice, which again takes us back to Mrs. Takata's instructions as well.

Mikao Usui wrote in the precepts, "Kokoro ni nenji," which also means deeply bearing in the mind/heart. When we bear the precepts deeply in our mind/heart, we have a state of mind of meditation. It is a state of mind in which we do not anger and worry, in which we are grateful for whatever comes our way, in which we are true to our way and our being, and in which we can be compassionate to ourselves and others. We can bring this state of mind of meditation with us in all we do: walking, shopping, hands-on healing, you name it... we can infuse our daily life with this state of mind of meditation.

Thus, as we can see, Mikao Usui's system is a system based on meditation practices which help us to lay bare the state of mind of meditation. And this state of mind of meditation is none other than the embodiment of the precepts. With the precepts as the foundation of the system of Reiki – words to live by – and as meditations themselves – a state of mind, principles to embody – we come full circle.

Chapter 20

Insights into Jōshin Kokyū Hō

Within Mikao Usui's teachings we find a meditation technique called jōshin kokyū hō. Jōshin kokyū hō is an essential meditation practice which is practiced throughout all levels of the system of Reiki, and therefore can be practiced for the rest of our lives.

But what is jōshin kokyū hō all about?
Translation:

Let's first look at the kanji of jōshin kokyū hō: 淨 jo means clear, pure, without taint or defilement, lucid
心 shin means heart, mind, essence, the mind as the principle of the universe, the enlightened mind
呼吸 kokyū means to exhale and inhale, breathing
法 hō means method, Dharma, principle

We therefore can translate jōshin kokyū hō in this way:

- The principle of pure mind/heart through breathing in and out.

- The method of realizing our enlightened mind through breathing in and out.

Thus when we practice jōshin kokyū hō on a daily basis for many years, we start to realize the principle that our mind/heart is as pure as the universe.

According to a Japanese Aikido practitioner, kokyū hō also means "work in perfect harmony."

We thus also can say that jōshin kokyū hō translates as "The principle of pure mind/heart through working in perfect harmony with the universe."

The practice:

1. Sit and gassho.
2. Place your hands in your lap, palms facing upwards.
3. With each in breath, feel a bright energy coming in through the nose and bring it down to the hara/tanden, just below your navel. When you do this, link the visual with the breath and the mind.
4. Feel the bright energy, the breath and the mind expanding through your body.
5. On the out breath, expand the bright energy, the breath and the mind out of the body, through your skin, out into infinity.
6. Repeat steps 3 through 5 until finished. Most important is that the mind is brought to the hara/tanden and that the mind expands through your body and into infinity. Visualizing the bright light and following the breath are an aid for this.

The practice of jōshin kokyū hō also resembles specific visualization meditation practices within Japanese esoteric Buddhism, such as the expansion visualizations (Jap: kakudai-ho), permeation visualizations (Jap: shinto-ho) and specific moon-disk visualizations (Jap: gachirin-kan).

Insights

The in breath into the nose and bringing the mind to the hara/ tanden is the first step of the practice. This is an important step as it helps us to bring our mind back into our body and under control, so that we do not get distracted by past, present and future. And as the hara/tanden is just below the navel it helps us to center and ground ourselves. But it is just the first step. If our mind stops at the hara/tanden we are missing the point of jōshin kokyū hō as jōshin kokyū hō is so much more! It goes far beyond simply grounding ourselves.

Zen master Takuan Soho describes very clearly in his book *The Unfettered Mind* why it is important not to stop at the hara/tanden:

> You should not place your mind within yourself. Bracing the mind in the body is something done only at the inception of training, when one is a beginner. But viewed from the highest standpoint of Buddhism, putting your mind just below the navel and not allowing it to wander is a low level of understanding, not a high one. It is at the level of discipline and training.

From a traditional meditation practice perspective, we can say that breathing into the hara and resting the mind there for a moment is a Shamatha (resting our mind on a single object) meditation practice. And expanding the mind out and leaving it wide open is a Vipashyana (clearly seeing that there is no "I") meditation practice. Combining both practices is a classical way of deeper teachings in Buddhism.

In his book, *Luminous Clarity: A Commentary on Karma Chagme's Union of Mahamudra and Dzogchen*, Khenchen Thrangu writes about some of these teachings and the benefit of combining these practices:

> However, if Vipashyana is cultivated without the accompanying cultivation of Shamatha, then that Vipashyana meditation becomes like a small boat that drifts in the stormy sea of our controlled mind.

It is only through cultivating Vipashyana properly endowed with Shamatha meditation that we can conquer the disturbing emotions.

Yes, it is important to rest our mind at the hara/tanden for grounding and centering, especially for a beginner. But within Mikao Usui's style of jōshin kokyū hō, we focus on the hara/tanden and expand the mind out into infinity. Bringing the mind to the hara/tanden is the foundation for expanding our mind into infinity.

In fact by naming it jōshin kokyū hō, Mikao Usui also is pointing why not to stop at the hara/tanden.

Koichi Tohei describes kokyū in his book *Aikido: The Coordination of Mind and Body for Self-defence* as: "Kokyu is, in plain words, the movement of your Ki or the movement of your body following Ki. If you have strong Kokyu, your body is filled with powerful Ki…" According to Koichi Tohei, kokyū is the movement of your Ki. And if this movement of Ki is strong, your whole body is filled with powerful Ki. Hence the expansion of the mind through your whole body during jōshin kokyū hō. If we only rest our mind on the hara/tanden, then our mind and energy will be stuck in one place. This is good for a beginner but if we want to go deeper, we need to expand it into infinity. The Ki needs to move through our body and not be stuck in one place.

Why do we need to expand our mind out into infinity? Because we need to realize that our mind is pure like the universe. The universe is infinite; there is no beginning or end. Thus through the daily practice of jōshin kokyū hō we start to slowly realize the principle that our mind is infinite like the universe. The universe doesn't stop at one point; it is infinitely open and expanded.

But this direct experience needs to be based on the hara/tanden; it is our starting point. If we do not expand from the hara/tanden, we will have a very hard time realizing this unification. Thus by connecting to the hara/tanden and expanding outwards into infinity, Mikao Usui killed two birds with one stone – grounding – centering and expanding into infinity. Realizing that our mind is always expanded like infinite space, the mind will not stop at one spot; it is just open. Hence the word open-mindedness; when we are open-minded we can accommodate everything and everyone. If our mind is stuck in one spot, we become narrow-minded and therefore have difficulty accommodating everything and everyone.

Zen master Takuan Soho points out in his book *The Unfettered Mind* why it is so important to expand the mind into infinity and not to focus on one point:

Considering that the Thousand-Armed Kannon has one thousand arms on its one body, if the mind stops at the one holding a bow, the other nine hundred and ninety-nine will be useless. It is because the mind is not detained at one place that all the arms are useful.

... the mind that does not stop at all is called immovable wisdom.

When our mind is not stopped at the hara/tanden but flows into infinite space, we are in a state of mind of immovable wisdom. This immovable wisdom doesn't mean our mind is focused on one spot, because if we focus on one spot we can get distracted and have to bring our mind back to this one spot again and again. Thus our mind is constantly moving from being distracted to bringing it back to one spot. Immovable wisdom is where our mind is wide open, and there is nothing to grasp in this wide-open space. Thus the mind is not moved by anything; hence, immovable wisdom. Thoughts come and go but as there is no grasping in this open space, they will dissolve all by themselves. No need to bring the mind back to anything, no need to do anything... just to be.

Even in other Buddhist teachings, they instruct us to do the same. Orgyen Chowang writes in his book, *The Pristine Mind*, "Do not make the scope of your meditation too narrow. Do not try to force your mind or your visual focus to stay in one spot or in one particular place." Orgyen Chowang explains this further:

If our meditation involves focusing on a single object, as in mindfulness meditation, then noises or other external distractions can take us away from that focus. But when our mind is not focused on any particular thing, then that noise just passes through our awareness without interrupting our meditation at all. When we try to hold our mind on one point by focusing on a particular object in meditation, then our awareness is not expansive but is listed to that one object. But when we are remaining in Pristine Mind and not holding our attention to any particular object, our awareness permeates the entire space we are in. All sound just passes through our awareness. After a certain point, when we are remaining in Pristine mind, sensory inputs from the external world do not affect us.

Mikao Usui also pointed this out by teaching the mantra hon sha ze sho nen in Okuden Reiki Level II. Hon sha ze sho nen literally translates as, "My original nature is a non-dual thought," but it also stands for "My original nature is Right Mind." Zen master Takuan Soho describes what Right Mind is: "The Right Mind is the mind that does not remain in one place. It is the mind that stretches throughout the entire universe." He also states that "When the Right Mind congeals and settles in one place it becomes what is called the confused mind."

A student of Mikao Usui wrote this: "Human consciousness can go anywhere in the universe in an instant. You must endeavor to develop your consciousness quickly and not to rely on the symbols for too long." This is very similar to what Takuan Soho is pointing out.

Hon sha ze sho nen and jōshin kokyū hō are two different

practices/paths to the same state of mind, a mind which is grounded and centered yet infinitely open and expanded. In this state, our mind can realize its non-dual nature. Or in other words, jōshin kokyū hō is about the realization that I am the universe and the universe is me.

A calm mind not tied to anything lets authentic wisdom appear. – Taisen Deshimaru, *Mushotoku Mind: The Heart of the Heart Sutra*

Thus as we can see, jōshin kokyū hō's deeper insight is that by practicing it on a daily basis, we can settle our mind from all our confused thoughts. When we do this, our mind can stretch and realize its oneness with the infinite universe so that authentic wisdom appears.

Chapter 21

Hatsurei hō – How to Reveal Your Hidden Ultimate Truth

The essence of any spiritual practice is to reveal the ultimate truth which is hidden deep inside of us. What is this truth? This truth is our true self. Different traditions have different names for it, but the essence is the same. Within the system of Reiki, the true self is symbolized by the word Reiki. Often Reiki is translated as "spiritual energy" but this spiritual energy is really our true self, our essence.

Mikao Usui left many clues as to what this spiritual energy really is, and many practices to help us to reveal it. One of the essential practices is called hatsurei hō, traditionally taught within Mikao Usui's teachings in Okuden Level II.

Let's take a deeper look at hatsurei hō and see what it is revealing.

The Japanese kanji for hatsurei hō is 発霊法. Hatsu 発 means to arise, to give birth, to reveal what is hidden or to emit.

Rei 霊 means spirit, soul or inconceivable spiritual ability.

Hō 法 means Dharma, ultimate truth or method.

We therefore could say that hatsurei hō means, "the ultimate truth to reveal our hidden inconceivable spiritual ability." This inconceivable spiritual ability is not hands-on healing; hands-on healing is simply a by-product of the spiritual practice. It is also not about seeing colors or feeling tingling or heat in our hands or body; these are also just by-products. This inconceivable spiritual ability is our true self/Reiki. It is inconceivable because we are not capable of imagining or mentally grasping this true self. This is why the teachers of old used poetry, paintings, metaphors and symbols to point out the true self. One of the ways Mikao Usui pointed out the inconceivable true self is through the precepts:

Do not be angry
Do not worry
Be grateful
Be true to your way and your being
Show compassion to yourself and others

It is only when we have revealed the ultimate truth of our true self that we are no longer angry and worried, that we are true to our way and our being, that we are grateful and compassionate to ourselves and others.

What is interesting to note is that hatsurei hō was traditionally taught in Okuden Level II, and that the word Okuden 奥伝 means hidden/inner teachings. Thus we can see that both Okuden and hatsurei hō are pointing to the same thing. They both reveal what is hidden deep inside of ourselves: our true self/Reiki.

Traditionally the symbols and mantras taught within the system of Reiki also were meditation practices to help us to reveal what was hidden inside of ourselves. However, over time those meditation practices have become more and more externalized. The more we externalize Reiki practice, the more we move away from looking inward and revealing our inconceivable spiritual ability, or true self.

Hatsurei hō also links to another practice within the system of Reiki. Hatsu also means to emit, which relates to the Shinpiden Level III symbol/mantra 大光明 which literally translates as "great bright light." When we are revealing our great bright light, we start to emanate or radiate this light through the whole world. We emanate love and compassion into the world; this is our ultimate truth.

Thus the more we practice hatsurei hō and meditate on the

symbols and mantras, the more we start to reveal our hidden ultimate truth, our true self, and the more we will be able to emanate healing into the world.

Chapter 22

Stoking the Fire of Practicing the System of Reiki

To stoke the fire of practice, we need to heat it up. The reason why we need to heat up the fire is so that we can burn away all our misconceptions, ignorance, anger, worries, fears, attachments, judgments, you name it.

This stoking is done through constant and right practice. And no, "constant" is not a typing error for "consistent."

Yes, indeed consistent practice is important. But constant practice means that practice is done not just when we sit on a meditation pillow, but throughout the whole day and night. We need to keep that fire burning.

Often we just practice for 10 minutes and then we forget about it. But what if we stay mindful of our practice throughout our day and even in the night? If we start to do that, we create a constant fire. And with this fire, we constantly are burning away all the stuff which obscures our true self.

Imagine a pot of water. If you want to boil the water, you want a strong and healthy flame; if the flame is weak and goes on and off all the time, the water never will boil. This is the same within the system of Reiki, or any practice for that matter. The main purpose of the system of Reiki is to remember our true self. But if our practice goes on and off and is not a healthy practice, then we never will remember our true self.

Why is remembering our true self so important? At the moment the world is not in a healthy state. But if we start to remember our true self, which emanates compassion and wisdom, then our whole world will start to change. Thus it is of utmost importance that we stoke the fires of practice before it is too late and our children inherit an earth which is polluted, destroyed, and with no compassion and love.

Right practice is bringing the practice inwards, into our own being, because it is only there that we will remember our true self. If we keep practicing externally and never want to deal with our own issues, we will not remember our true self.

Right practice is therefore meditating on the precepts, meditating on the symbols and mantras, practicing the meditation practices like jōshin kokyū hō and hatsurei hō, practicing hands-on healing on ourselves as meditation, and being in a meditative state of mind while we perform and "receive" reiju/initiation/attunement.

But as stated before, if we only do this occasionally, then the water will not boil.

The quickest way to stoke the fire and boil the water is to go to the roots of all our issues. And that is our mind. Mikao Usui pointed this out as well within the precepts:

Do not anger
Do not worry
Be grateful
Practice diligently
Show compassion to yourself and others

The precepts are about the root of all our issues; they are the spiritual medicine, and they are about the mind. Thus if we really want to stoke the fire or embrace the system of Reiki with right practice, we have to go straight to the mind. We cannot always chant a mantra day and night, we cannot always practice hatsurei hō day and night, we cannot always do hands-on healing day and night. But we can place our mind in the right state of mind day and night. This state of mind is the mind of no anger, no worry, being grateful and compassionate. And if we practice this diligently, day and night, day in and day out, we create a healthy fire which will bring the water to boil in no time. This in turn means that we start to remember our true self in no time. And this will have a tremendous ripple effect throughout the world.

Chapter 23

We Always Can Go Deeper

Often, after finishing a Reiki class, we think that is it. We have gotten a certificate and now we don't have to go deeper.

But the system of Reiki is so much more than just taking a class. Classes are just the beginning. Within a class the teacher not only explains the essence of the system, but also tries to facilitate change so that the students have a direct experience of their true self/Reiki.

In fact even Shinpiden Reiki III is not the end of the line but rather the start. For at this level we start to see and understand that it is a lifelong journey. That life becomes practice and practice becomes life. This comes from having the direct experience that the precepts can be incorporated into all we do. Not just when we do some hands-on healing on ourselves or on others, but in every moment in our lives.

By setting the intent before we start out on a class that we want to rediscover our true self, to bring inner happiness into our lives, we create a clear path. If there is no clear intent, we walk around aimlessly. It's like if we want to start walking the Appalachian Trail, we need to have a clear intent of where to start and where to go. Otherwise we just walk around in circles.

The classes are in reality an initial experience, where we start to see and feel what is possible. But this initial experience is not yet a full-blown experience which is infused in our daily life. After the initial experience of taking a class, now we need to practice diligently. Within the system of Reiki, these practices consist of meditating on the precepts, meditating on the symbols and mantras, meditation practices like jōshin kokyū hō, practicing hands-on healing as a form of meditation, and performing Reiju or "receiving" Reiju as a form of support for our meditation practice. The more we practice these meditation practices, the deeper we go. The deeper we go, the more we start to integrate the precepts into our daily life so that all we do becomes infused with love and compassion.

This is why we always can go deeper; we always can be more compassionate and loving. The real aim is to be so compassionate that we can embrace the whole universe with love – or in other words, that we have realized that we are the universe and the universe is us.

Imagine what could happen if you could offer a client or student the whole universe? Just imagine...

But right now most of us, including me, cannot do this because of our attachments, fears, worries, anger, you name it. Thus, the more we practice, the more we let go of our anger, worries, and fears, the more grateful and compassionate we become, and the more we can offer ourselves and others.

So if you begin to offer yourself the gift of diligent practice now, imagine what you could offer over time? Just imagine...

Chapter 24

Self-Practice and Self-Care Within the System of Reiki

Self-practice is in reality also practicing for and with others; we cannot divide them – self is others and others is self.

Within the system of Reiki we often hear the terms self-care and self-practice. Most of the time they point towards the aspect of hands-on healing on ourselves, and hands-on healing on ourselves is a wonderful aspect of self-care.

However, there are many more tools within the system of Reiki which also are techniques for self-care and self-practice.

The Precepts
Do not anger
Do not worry
Be grateful
Be true to your way and your being
Show compassion to yourself and others

By meditating on the precepts, we start to gain insights into why we get angry and worry, why we are not grateful and not being true to our way and our being, and why we are not compassionate to ourselves and others. These insights will help us to let go of our anger and worry, and therefore we become more grateful, true to our way and our being and more compassionate. All of this will trigger an inner happiness and openness within ourselves; thus, it is self-care and self-practice. By meditating on the precepts, we are healing our confused monkey mind.

Mantras and Symbols

Traditionally the mantras and symbols were utilized within the system of Reiki as meditation tools. We focus our mind on the symbol and we chant the mantra. By doing this we start to become more focused; we slowly stop following our thoughts to the past, present, and future. The less we follow our thoughts to the past, present, and future the more open and relaxed we become. This in turn starts to create a more open flow of energy through our whole body, because an open expanded mind means an open and expanded free-flowing energy. Since energy follows the mind, the calmer our mind is, the calmer our energy will be. The more open-minded we become, the more open our energy will be until we become so open that we are now as expanded as – and one with – the universe. Thus we can see that the mantras and symbols also are tools for self-care and self-practice.

Meditations

Within the system of Reiki there also are specific meditation practices like jōshin kokyū hō and hatsurei hō. These practices help us again to calm our mind. The calmer our mind is, the calmer our body and energy becomes.

Current scientific research shows that meditation practices in which we focus on our breath or a mantra, or we contemplate, are very beneficial for healing ourselves. Science now tells us that meditation practice reduces blood pressure, lessens heart and brain problems, strengthens our immune system, and helps us to become less anxious and depressed. Thus we now also can start to see that these meditation practices within the system of Reiki are self-care and self-practice.

Reiju/Initiation/Attunements

The Reiju is yet another form of self-care and self-practice. By performing a Reiju on someone else, the teacher enters a state of expanded consciousness in which she will try as much as possible to remember the union with all that is. By doing this, the teacher will start to feel her whole body becoming more at ease; maybe she will even experience a feeling that her body is not there at all. This in turn will trigger a free-flowing energy through her whole being, which in essence is healing in nature. Thus Reiju also is self-care and self-practice.

Hands-on Healing

As stated before, many people when they mention self-care or self-practice are talking about doing hands-on healing on themselves. However, as we now can see, all the other tools within Mikao Usui's teachings are also practices for self-care and self-practice. Thus if we are asked what we are doing, it would be much clearer and to the point to say that we are doing hands-on healing instead of self-care or self-practice. Because when we say self-care or self-practice, we also can mean that we are meditating on the precepts, meditating with the symbols and mantras, practicing the meditation techniques like jōshin kokyū hō and hatsurei hō, or performing a reiju/initiation/attunement. The clearer we are in saying what we are doing, the clearer our practice becomes, and thus, the clearer our point is to the wider public. So when we are clear about our practice within the system of Reiki, and we talk about our practice, people will know what we are talking about.

Self is Others and Others is Self

Now we come to the juicy part, self is others and others is self. We cannot separate them in our practice because on the deepest level of healing, wholeness, we are all interconnected. One of the precepts is: "show compassion to yourself and others"; Mikao Usui was already pointing out that self is others and others is self. But what is compassion to ourselves? Real compassion to ourselves is trying to remember our true self – Reiki – because that is the deepest form of healing. However, by remembering our true self we start to rediscover our inner wisdom and compassion, which we can utilize to show compassion to others. What is compassion to others? Helping others to remember their true self.

Thus the best intent for when we practice the techniques for ourselves is that we do it to remember our true self so that we can help others to remember their true self.

> The spiritual level of the practitioner directly reflects the effect of Reiki. In a sense, the more you are enlightened, the more the effectiveness of Reiki enhances. The more you practice Reiki for saving others, the brighter your innate light shines to drive away clouds covering your mind. I think this is the quintessence of Reiki. I hope that Frans Stiene's way of understanding Reiki spreads in the world to enlighten those who practice Reiki based on a superficial understanding of the tradition.
> – Takeda Hakusai Ajari

While our intent is not to "practice Reiki for saving others" from an egoistic standpoint, our practice helps us to become more compassionate to ourselves and others, to experience and embrace the interconnectedness of all. In this way, we can help ourselves and others move ever closer to healing and wholeness, to our true self.

Chapter 25

How to Stop Being Uncomfortable with Ourselves

All the practices within the system of Reiki are there foremost to help ourselves to become more comfortable within our own hearts and minds. However, these practices are not always that easy as they can stir up stuff. This is one of the reasons why most of the elements within the system of Reiki have become so externalized over the years, as we do not like to look deeply within ourselves. It scares us.

These practices take time. It is like trying to train a wild horse; the wild horse represents our confused mind. It takes a lot of effort and patience to train a wild horse and sometimes we fall off the horse and hurt ourselves. We stir up emotions, things we do not want to look at: fear, worry, anger, you name it. But if we want to help others, then it is of utmost importance that we start to tame our own confused mind first.

The more we do this, the more we start to be comfortable within ourselves. But what does that mean? It means that we start to accept ourselves for who we are with all our pain, discomfort, joy, issues, and attachments. We start to become friends with ourselves again instead of saying things like, "I am not good enough," or "I have this or that issue and therefore I am not pretty enough," and so on. I call this "being naked" with yourself. Being naked is about accepting yourself completely, without judging or labelling. It is letting go of criticizing ourselves. The precept "show compassion to yourself" is pointing this out.

When we stop labelling and judging ourselves, we reach a state of mind of stillness. But as we are not used to being still, we start to label, distinguish, and judge again to create some internal entertainment. This internal dialogue analyzes everything, and that is why we feel so tired. If our minds are busy all the time, we are never still. In this way, we are depleting our energy.

But if we cannot be still within ourselves, how can we be still when we are with others?

This is one of the main reasons we keep labelling, judging, and distinguishing during a hands-on healing session, rather than being in a state of mind of stillness and openness. We find it uncomfortable to be still. We want to keep busy analyzing, because most of the time we are scared of what will happen when we are in a state of mind of stillness. The precept "show compassion to others" also points out this stillness.

The Reiki precepts can remind us to cultivate this state of stillness:

Do not be angry
Do not worry
Be grateful
Be true to your way and your being
Show compassion to yourself and others

We can see that compassion to others is the last precept. Why? Because we first need to become comfortable within ourselves to create this still, open, naked state of mind. When we are compassionate to others, there is no judging, labelling and distinguishing going on, just stillness.

Let's take a closer look at some of the teachings within the system of Reiki and see how they point towards being comfortable within ourselves, so that we feel we can be still.

Jōshin kokyū hō, an essential meditation taught in Shoden Reiki Level I, is about bringing our mind into the hara/tanden, an energy center just below our navel. We do this so that we become centered and still. When our mind is focused on one point, the hara/tanden, then we do not become distracted by our own internal busyness; thus we become more still and accepting of ourselves.

The first symbol taught in Okuden Reiki Level II is doing exactly the same thing. Traditionally you would meditate on it to become more comfortable with yourself and not be distracted by labelling, judging, and distinguishing, which is our constant internal dialogue. Where are our minds normally? All over the place, thinking about the past, present, and future. Now look at the first symbol and trace it with your mind; where is your mind going? Inwards!!! Yes, now imagine doing this again and again and again. What starts to happen? We get less distracted and thus we start to accept ourselves more and more. In turn, this will help us to get less distracted when we perform hands-on healing on others too; we finally can just be with our clients.

If we look closely at all the other tools within Mikao Usui's teachings we can start to see the same thing. They are all there to help us to become more comfortable within ourselves, and therefore with the world around us. Now we can be still – free – with no more labelling, judging, and distinguishing.

Chapter 26

Reiki and Depression

As stated previously, according to the World Health Organization, more than 350 million people around the world suffer from depression. The WHO website states that depression is on the rise and describes some of its symptoms as reduced energy, leading to diminished activities and a loss of enjoyment.

The system of Reiki offers many practices to combat the loss of enjoyment and the feeling of having no energy to be involved in daily activities. So practicing the system of Reiki is a great tool for dealing with depression.

One of the reasons we feel a lack of energy during depression is because the energy needed to participate in daily life is eaten up by fear, worry, and anger. In this state, we also lose our inner joy, our inner happiness. Constant fear, worry, and anger leave us tired and depleted. Therefore, one of the main aspects is to replenish our energy so that we can start to feel our inner joy again.

One of the most important meditation practices within the system of Reiki is jōshin kokyū hō, a meditation practice in which we focus on and bring our breath into the hara/tanden, just below our navel. This energy center is our center, our foundation, our inner battery. By mindfully breathing into this area, slowly we start to replenish our energy in this battery and at the same time we start to feel more grounded and centered. By grounding and centering ourselves we start to move away from our monkey mind, and therefore we start to soften our grip on fear, worry, and anger. This in turn gradually helps us to let go of our depressive state of mind.

Another practice is the chanting of mantras. Mantra means protection for the mind. Chanting protects our mind from straying into fear, worry, and anger, and therefore mantras are a great tool for softening our depression. Another aspect of chanting mantras, if we do it correctly, is that the sound starts to vibrate through our whole being. This gives us a pleasurable feeling, a feeling of inner warmth and contentment. These feelings help us to feel more love and compassion for ourselves and thus, we can start to lose our grip on our depression.

Compassion is another element which can help us with our depression, specifically being compassionate to others. Showing compassion to others is a great way of letting go of our own self-pity and we can do this by helping others. In doing this, we start to move away from the focus on ourselves and on our own self-pity. The ultimate aim of the system of Reiki is to rediscover our innate great bright light; this light is the light of playfulness, open and expanded, full of joy and passion for life. When we rediscover this light, our depression will melt and vanish like snow in the sun. But this is not always easy to accomplish; it takes time and effort. So be patient with yourself. Practice diligently, and find a good teacher who can teach you how to empower yourself so that you slowly over time can start to rediscover your own inner great bright light of happiness.

Chapter 27

How to Cope as an Empath

Empathy means that we sense and feel what the other person is experiencing; we empathize with them. Empathy can be a great asset as it can help us to feel and see what someone is going through, which in turn will help us to understand the person better. However, it also can have its drawbacks. We can be too empathic, and if we start to experience the suffering of the person directly, this can lead to empathy distress.

If we feel we are entering the state of mind of empathy distress, there are great techniques and insights to help us. By practicing these techniques and contemplating these insights, we can learn how to cope as an empathic person.

Weeble Wobble

The first and foremost important practice is to start to feel more grounded and centered. This centered feeling helps us not to get too overwhelmed with empathy distress. Try to breathe deeply into your hara/tanden, which is an energetic center just below your navel; it is our foundation. Remember the Weeble Wobble? Weebles Wobble but don't fall. Why? Because they are solid at the bottom yet they are flexible. We have to be like a Weeble Wobble. Often we may get pushed over and simply lie down, feeling too overwhelmed to retain our footing or regain our balance. But if our energy and focus is strong at the hara/tanden, we become like a Weeble Wobble; we come back up straightaway after we experience a deep sense of empathy.

Grounding

We need even more grounding. In our current world we are so

in our heads that this can amplify the empathic distress state of mind. Computers, phones, TV, intellectualizing everything – we are busy in our head constantly while the focus on our center, our grounding, the earth, is not being promoted. The below grounding method is – besides Tip 1, breathing and focusing on the hara/tanden – one of the fastest and easiest ways of grounding that I have practiced.

Lie with your back flat on the floor, with your feet against the wall. This means that your legs are not on the floor, your knees are slightly bent, and your feet are against the wall at a height that is comfortable for you. Place your hands above your head and now very consciously slowly push the energy all the way down with your hands to your hara/tanden just below your navel. As soon as your hands reach the hara/tanden, place them physically on this area and apply a slight pressure with your feet. You do not push yourself away from the wall, just a slight pressure. This pressure will help the mind go to the feet, which in turn helps the energy go to the feet. Energy follows the mind. Release the slight pressure on the feet and bring your hands back to above your head again. Repeat the whole procedure again. Do this for about 10 times.

Compassion in action

Try to mix in compassion with your empathy. Empathy is suffering with the person, while compassion is the state of mind in which we want to help the other person to overcome their suffering. When we start to look at ways of helping others, this takes the focus away from ourselves; hence compassion in action slowly starts to soften our empathic distress. However, to be more compassionate we need to let go of our own anger, fear, worries, and attachments. This means that we need to apply how to be a Weeble Wobble and more grounding.

Be open like space

This is one of the hardest elements to understand if we are extremely empathic. The ultimate aim is to have a state of mind which is open and expanded like space. A spacious mind doesn't hold onto anything, is not disturbed by anything, and is not hurt by anything. As our mind and energy are interlinked, a spacious mind therefore also means a spacious energy. Our mind and energy have a huge effect on our physical well-being; thus a spacious mind/energy also means a spacious sense in our physical body. All of this spaciousness means that our empathic feelings do not stick in our mind, energy, and body. This is the spaciousness of our true self, our essence in which we have let go of the "I." When there is no "I," then there is also no "I" who experiences any empathic distress. At this stage we can stop saying: "But I am an empath; I pick up things."

As you can see, this is why being open like space is not that easy. It takes dedication and practice, but in the end it is well worth it. What a freedom and sense of relief it brings.

Practice daily

Because we are so used to being empathic that it has become a habit, the previous tips really can only start to work when we practice these breathing and meditation practices on a daily basis. In the beginning, spend at least 10 to 20 minutes doing these daily practices; in doing this, we slowly start to change our mindset and our energetic behavior patterns. After a while, start to increase your daily practice to at least 45 minutes every day.

All of this might take weeks, months, or years, depending on our current state of mind. Therefore, mix in a bit of patience with the practice; that way we do not get angry or worried when we feel these breathing and meditation practices are not working as quickly as we might like or expect them to. If we remind ourselves to let go of expectations and just be where we are at any given moment, we will create more room within ourselves to focus on consistent practice. In doing this – releasing expectations and attachments and practicing daily our grounding, breathing, compassion, spaciousness, patience – we will find it easier to cope with life as an empath.

Part 3

Hands-on Healing

Chapter 28

Hands-on Healing as Meditation

Hands-on healing on ourselves and others is in essence a form of moving meditation.

But for hands-on healing to become meditation a few factors need to be at play.

Often when we perform hands-on healing on ourselves we fall asleep. Thus we cannot really call it a meditation anymore because there is no clarity and focus, and we are not mindful.

Often when we perform hands-on healing on others we start to get sidetracked by our thought process. We get carried away by the past, present, and future. Maybe we get carried away by what our senses are experiencing; we start to follow the experience so to speak, instead of being mindful. Thus if our senses get carried away by our thought process, hands-on healing also ceases to be meditation.

When someone performs a hands-on healing session on us, this also can become a meditation. But again, oftentimes we either fall asleep or we get carried away by all our senses. But if we are mindful during our session, then hands-on healing for ourselves, performed by someone else, also can become meditation.

The first miracle brought about by mindfulness is your own presence, your real presence. With this energy dwelling in you, you become completely alive. When the energy of mindfulness is dwelling in you, Buddha is dwelling in you. The energy of mindfulness is the energy of Buddha. It is the equivalent of the Holy Spirit. Where the Holy Spirit is, there is also understanding, life, healing, and compassion. Where mindfulness is, true life, solidity, freedom, and healing also manifest. We all have the

ability to generate this energy of mindfulness.
– Thich Nhat Hanh, *You Are Here: Discovering the Magic of the Present Moment*

When we are mindful during hands-on healing, whether we perform it on ourselves or on someone else, or if someone else is performing it on us, hands-on healing becomes meditation.

Why is it so essential for hands-on healing to become meditation? Because when we are in a state of mind of meditation, we are mindful. Being mindful creates an open expanded state of mind in which the energy can flow freely through us. This free-flowing energy in turn can take us to a level of healing much deeper than if we get sidetracked by all our senses during a hands-on healing session.

When we start to move into a space of meditation during hands-on healing, our energy becomes more free-flowing because it is not getting caught up by daily issues which we may be thinking about.

As Thich Nhat Hanh states: "The energy of mindfulness is the energy of Buddha." Or in other words, the energy of mindfulness is the energy of the whole cosmos.

Most of the time our mind is all over the place, distracted by the past, present, and future, distracted by all our senses. In this distracted state, we are not realizing our full potential of being the energy of the cosmos. As energy follows the mind, it is therefore essential to be mindful during hands-on healing so that it becomes a moving meditation practice. Wouldn't it be amazing if we could offer someone the whole cosmos instead of our confused monkey mind? With mindfulness, with a hands-on-healing session that is a moving meditation, we can.

This of course also is explained within the precepts; the precepts tell us to be mindful. The word precept can also mean instruction; thus the precepts instruct us how to perform a hands-on healing session in the mindful state that the precepts themselves help us to cultivate. In fact, all the other tools within the system of Reiki also point this out. Therefore the deeper we go within the practice of the system of Reiki, the more mindful we become and the more hands-on healing becomes a meditation practice. The deeper we go, the more we remember our union with the cosmos and the more energy will flow freely through us, helping healing to occur.

Chapter 29

Working With…

As practitioners or teachers we often say: "I am doing hands-on healing on someone," or "I am working on someone."

But "working on" implies that the practitioner "does something to" the client and the client just has to lie back and doesn't need to do anything! However, as we are not the healers but rather the facilitators, the client needs to be open and have a willingness to heal themselves. Their openness and willingness to heal themselves is the trigger for real healing to take place, because in essence we can only heal ourselves.

Therefore a better way of saying this would be, "I am doing hands-on healing with someone" or "I am working with someone." Saying "with" rather than "on" illustrates the partnership of practitioner and client.

Hands-on healing is like a meditative dance and, as we all know, it takes two to tango. The way we word things in our practice is thus very important. Words carry energy and energy needs to be empowering and not disempowering. Working together with our clients empowers us both, and thus creates a beautiful dance of healing.

Chapter 30

Mind/heart and Hands-on Healing

I often get asked the question from Reiki teachers and students alike: Why do some practitioners and/or teachers have more energy coming out of their hands than others?

Some even go further than that and ask: Why do some practitioners and/or teachers emanate more energy from their whole being than others?

When some of these practitioners put their hands on someone it feels like a tingling moving through the body, like electricity. Or a heat, warmth, or light emanating from their body/being.

This greater amount of energy is really only possible through personally practicing the meditations taught within the traditional Japanese system of Reiki.

Mikao Usui's Students

A note from Mikao Usui's student states this:

> We humans hold the Great Reiki that fills the Great Universe. The higher we raise the vibration of our own being, the stronger the Reiki we have inside will be.

Another student of Mikao Usui, Kaiji Tomita, wrote this in his book *Reiki To Jinjutsu: Tomita Ryu Teate Ryoho* about hatsurei hō, a Japanese Reiki meditation technique:

> Sit in the seiza position and gassho with the objective to gather/ concentrate the energy from the heart into the palms of the

hands. Hold the hands together without using force from the arms or the shoulders. Drop the shoulders and clasp the hands, joining the fingers lightly, and feel the alignment of the posture... If you have followed the previous steps and stayed focused on the palms of your hands, they will likely start to feel warm. This is what (Tomita Ryu) calls reiha (Jap: wave of rei). It describes the tingling sensation that is comparable to an electrical current. The heat created and the wave of rei are what constitute spiritual energy. Even if the sensations are weak at first, they should become stronger as you keep concentrating.

Hatsurei hō literally translates as "Generating a greater amount of spirit."

By looking at some of Mikao Usui's students we can see that we need to meditate to let the energy/Reiki come out from within.

Mind/heart

Hatsurei hō and other elements within the Japanese system of Reiki point towards a very important location, our mind/heart.

Within hatsurei hō we place our hands in gassho in front of the heart center, and within Okuden Reiki Level II we find the mantra HSZSN. Within the kanji of HSZSN is the kanji of Nen 念 and within this we also can see the kanji of Shin/Kokoro 心. They call Shin/Kokoro the radical of Nen; a radical is a clue to the origin of the kanji and also to the general meaning.

Shin/Kokoro means mind/heart, wholeheartedness, the enlightened mind, essence, the mind as the principle of the universe, center, core, etc. In these traditional teachings there is no division between the heart and our mind; they are seen as one. So why is Shin/Kokoro the key to generating a greater amount or stronger flow of energy?

Traditionally the mind/heart moves the blood and ki/energy.

It is in the mind/heart center that the earth and heavenly energy unite. When these unite, we gain harmony between the two opposite elements, therefore creating harmony within our own energy. This in turn creates a greater flow of energy.

But to unite heaven and earth energy within our mind/heart center we first need to become earth and heavenly energy. This is taught within the traditional Japanese Reiki teachings in Okuden Level II, in which the first two symbols and mantras represent earth and heavenly energy. But we need to become them, not just intend it; this is a very important part of Mikao Usui's traditional way of teaching.

This union also creates an openness, like an open welcoming heart or like an open mind which doesn't get angry or worried when something happens. The more open we become, the more energy emanates from our whole being. And the deeper we go into this openness, the more we start to remember our own innate great bright light. Or in other words, when our mind/heart becomes clear and open, our true self is revealed.

When our mind/heart center becomes clearer and clearer, we also start to feel a greater amount of energy flowing out of our hands; this is also due to the heart meridian through which the energy flows. The heart meridian flows upwards from the heart into the lungs, outward into the armpits and then down into the arms, to the hands and into the little fingers. Therefore, the clearer the heart, the clearer the heart meridians, the more energy will flow out of your hands.

This is why hatsurei hō is such an excellent meditation practice, to purify the heart meridian and create an openness within our mind/heart and therefore generate a greater flow of energy into our hands and being.

Your Heart Is Not in It

Have you ever heard the saying, "Your heart is not in it"?

The deeper meaning of this saying is that when our mind/heart is not in the practice of hands-on healing or a reiju/initiation/attunement then we are not connecting the practice with our true self, from our core so to speak; thus there is not much energy flowing. The more we perform these practices from our mind/heart, the more energy will flow through our whole being. But this, of course, takes time as we first need to purify the mind/heart center and unite the earth and heavenly energy.

Openness Is Like Space

When our mind/heart is open we become like space, no beginning or end, completely open, unified with the universe. This also means we start to become more open-minded, letting go of anger and worry – because in this open space nothing sticks. Like a bird who flies in the spacious open sky, it leaves no trace at all. And this will be the same with our mind/heart. We leave no trace; something comes up in our mind/heart but we do not cling. So no trace is left.

When we look into space we see nothing at all because in reality we cannot see space. Therefore, by becoming like space we are free of all projections; nothing clings to space and space has enough openness to accommodate everything.

This, in turn, will generate a tremendous amount of compassion; or in other words, we can say that openness and spaciousness is compassion. This is why Mikao Usui has the precept "Show compassion to yourself and others"; he is pointing out this open mind/heart state. Because if we want to be compassionate to all sentient beings, we need to be able to accommodate everything. And this can only happen when our mind/heart is free from clinging.

Our Hands

So how do hands-on healing and openness work together? If our mind/heart becomes more open and spacious, then we start to realize that working with the hands is only the first step of the system of Reiki. At this stage we start to Be Reiki and the energy within our being is so open and spacious that it travels and emanates through our whole being. Here we can just sit opposite each other and let the healing happen all by itself.

Human consciousness can go anywhere in the universe in an instant.
– Note from a student of Mikao Usui

Anshin Ritsumei

Many Japanese Reiki teachers say that Mikao Usui achieved Anshin Ritsumei/Enlightenment. Anshin means: mind/heart in peace. So, again we see that Mikao Usui's teachings point towards an open mind/heart.

Chapter 31

The Precepts are the Foundation for Hands-on Healing

We all can do hands-on healing; it is in fact very easy. Just place your hands on (or near) yourself or someone else and there you go! Right?

Well, yes. But…

Mikao Usui instructed us with the precepts on how to perform hands-on healing. Remember, the word precepts also means instructions. So let's look at the precepts and see how they actually instruct us, and see how this will change our hands-on healing session.

> The precepts are…
> Do not anger
> Do not worry
> Be grateful
> Be true to your way and your being
> Show compassion to yourself and others

If we perform hands-on healing with anger, our mind is turbulent. Therefore, our energy is turbulent as well, and not as calm as when we have let go of our anger.

If we are worried, then our mind is distracted. Therefore, our energy is distracted as well, and not as focused as when we have let go of worry.

If we perform a session and we are not grateful – maybe the client says something, or maybe some pain in our head has not dissipated – then maybe we get worried and angry. This in turn leads to an agitated mind and agitated energy. By being grateful, our mind and energy become stable, open, and calm.

If we are not true to our way and our true self, we are scattered. And if we try to be true to someone else's way, this might cause issues and thus we will get worried and angry again. But if we are true to our way and our true self, our sessions flow organically, free from anger and worry.

If we perform a session without compassion to ourselves and others, instead we may infuse it with anger and worry again. Compassion is about letting go of all of that; in fact the deepest form of compassion is seeing that there is no giver, gift and receiver, seeing things as completely open like space. Thus in this spaciousness of compassion, our mind and energy are also spacious with no restriction; they move with pure flow, which means we are free from anger and worry.

As you can see, the basic form of hands-on healing is very easy but to go into the inner heart of hands-on healing, we need to infuse it with the precepts. When we infuse hands-on healing with the precepts, we get a very different kind of session. We get a session which is free from anger and worry, a session in which we are in a state of mind of being grateful, true to our way and our being, and compassionate.

This is why Mikao Usui introduced the precepts. Because without the instructions within the precepts, we lose the foundation of hands-on healing. And without the instructions within the precepts, we not only lose the foundation of hands-on healing, but we also lose the foundation of the whole system of Reiki.

Chapter 32

Hands-on Healing is a Manifestation of Compassion

When we start to integrate the precepts into our daily life, we start to feel more and more compassionate to ourselves and others. This is because we are slowly letting go of our anger, worry, and fears. We start to become more and more grateful, organic, and compassionate.

The compassion which is being reawakened is our own innate compassion; it is the warmth from our inner great bright light which we are laying bare through our daily meditation practice. This compassionate light is full of love and energy.

When this starts to happen, we start to investigate how we can utilize this compassionate warmth and energy. For most of us, the first point of call is our hands because we use our hands to touch, feel, extend, embrace, you name it. Plus we often can feel this compassionate energy in our hands because the heart meridians flow through our arms and into our hands.

So what do we do? We want to place our hands on ourselves or on others as an act of compassion.

When we place our hands on ourselves, we are in fact saying to our own being: "I love you, all is well. I know I am in pain and discomfort, but that is okay. Relax, open up, it is as it is." This kind of act of hands-on healing as a manifestation of compassion also helps us to become intimate with ourselves again. This in turn helps us to heal and open up to the universal flow of love.

And we can place our hands on someone else as an extension of our compassion, to support them so that they can say the same thing to themselves. Now we start to feel intimate with them, so that the universal flow of love and compassion can support them in their healing.

However, when we go deeper and deeper into our practice, we start to have the direct experience that the essential element we are touching with is not our hands, but our mind/heart. Because if our mind/heart of compassion is not in our touch, then our hands may be filled with warmth, but our touch is empty of love.

Chapter 33

Holding Space During a Hands-on Healing Session

Heather Plett wrote a wonderful article called, "What it Really Means to Hold Space for Someone." Here is a quote from the article:

> What does it mean to "hold space" for someone else? It means that we are willing to walk alongside another person in whatever journey they're on without judging them, making them feel inadequate, trying to fix them, or trying to impact the outcome. When we hold space for other people, we open our hearts, offer unconditional support, and let go of judgment and control.

How does holding space therefore relate to hands-on healing?

If we hold space for someone during a hands-on healing session, then we need to let go of any outcome. As soon as we have an idea that the pain needs to be gone or that an emotional issue needs to be resolved, then we are holding on to a certain outcome. And therefore, as we are holding on to this certain outcome, we are not holding space. Holding space means letting go of trying to fix our client. As soon as we try to fix our client, our ego is in the way and therefore we are not holding space.

Holding space during a session therefore also means that we need to let go of judging, labelling, and distinguishing because as soon as we are doing that, we also are coming from the ego. And in holding on to a judgment, label, or a distinction, again we are letting go of holding space. For example, some teachers teach that you need to use a specific symbol to heal an emotional issue. But that too is about judging, labelling, and distinguishing. Because as soon as we do this, we are trying to impact the outcome.

In reality the precepts of the system of Reiki are instructing us how to hold space:

Do not anger
Do not worry
Be grateful
Be true to your direct experience
Show compassion to yourself and others

If we judge, label, and distinguish during a session, we have moved away from being grateful and showing compassion. Real gratefulness and compassion is beyond judging, labelling and distinguishing what is good or bad, what is hot or cold. Real gratefulness and compassion is only possible when we open our mind/heart and step into the space of our inner great bright light, which is a state of non-duality, a state beyond judging, labelling and distinguishing.

Therefore a real practitioner and teacher will just hold their client in the light. And this is the real essence of holding space. This inner great bright light is the light of the universe which is like space: no beginning and end, and therefore devoid of judging, labelling and distinguishing.

The system of Reiki is first and most of all a spiritual practice so that we can let go of the ego and move beyond judging, labelling and distinguishing, so that we can properly hold space for our clients. Thus to be able to hold space for a client, first we need to rediscover how to hold space for ourselves.

If I do not know how to hold space for myself, how can I hold space for my client? When we know how to hold space for ourselves, then we know what it means to open our hearts, offer unconditional support, and let go of judgment and control. When we know how to hold space for ourselves, we truly can hold space for others when we share a hands-on healing session with them, because we are sharing our hearts, our support, and our light.

Chapter 34

Hands-on Healing in Hospitals

More and more, the system of Reiki is being introduced within hospitals and medical settings around the world.

But for a practitioner it is not always that easy to work in these kinds of environments. So here are a few essential tips to help you on your way.

Stay centered

Working in a medical setting, many things happen which can throw us off our center, losing our groundedness. Emergencies, people with trauma, crying, feeling pain, dying – you name it. All of these things can throw us off balance; this is why the practice of jōshin kokyū hō is so important. This is a deep breathing meditation practice in which you focus on your hara/tanden, an energy point just below your navel. This is your center.

Remember the Weeble Wobble? "Weebles wobble but they don't fall down." That is because the weight is in the bottom of the Weeble which makes it stable. The more our own focus is on our hara/tanden, the more stability we gain. The more we practice jōshin kokyū hō – on a daily basis – the more grounded we will become. We can move freely, but we do not fall over in distress or sink into the emotional difficulties of being in a hospital.

The moment we face a crisis, we learn whether or not our inner strength is sufficiently developed to carry us through our difficulties.
– Tarthang Tulku, *Openness Mind*

Don't label, judge, or distinguish

Letting go of labelling, judging, and distinguishing will help you to become more open. When we see a client in a hospital and we label them as sick, there already is an unbalanced "us and them" element at play. We are healthy; they are sick. For a treatment to be beneficial we need to create harmony, harmony between us and our client. I often hear from people who have cancer that they feel they are seen as "that cancer person," while they feel they are just a "person who has cancer." By not labelling, judging or distinguishing we start to see everybody as equal.

Most of your clients also are not interested in diagnosis; they just want to get better. So let go of labelling, judging, and distinguishing, and just be with them. Being with them frees up the energy within your own mind and therefore creates a more open space for healing to take place.

> As the senses communicate information to the mind, the mind begins to make decisions, which involve judgment, concepts, and dualities, that then create separateness and conflict.
> – Tarthang Tulku, *Openness Mind*

Be flexible

Often we learn that treatments need to be an hour long or even longer, but in hospital settings we do not always have the time to spend that long with a client. Sometimes all you have is 10 or 20 minutes. This doesn't mean that your session will not be beneficial; it is just that you have to be more flexible. Often we like to make our hands-on healing session complicated, but again, a hospital setting is not the place for this. Thus we have to be flexible so that we can let go of our "normal" way of doing things. Flexibility can only happen when we are more open-minded and less restricted with our practices. No need for specific hand positions, no need to wave your hand around, draw symbols or say mantras: keep it simple.

As we become more open, we experience a sense of liberation and the energy is free to flow within us.
– Tarthang Tulku, *Openness Mind*

Release expectation

When we see people in hospitals we might have lots of expectations of "making" them better. Expectations can become an obstacle because when these expectations are not met we start to worry or get angry. We worry that our sessions are not good enough; we get angry because the person is still sick. Expectation creates a breeding ground for all sorts of distractions. So let go of expectations: just be free and open.

It is important not to strive to attain any particular experience – so relax without distraction.
– Tarthang Tulku, *Openness Mind*

Embrace compassion

By far, the most important element for working in a hospital is compassion; it is one of the essential precepts within the system of Reiki. Compassion is the last precept because we only can be truly compassionate when we have let go of our anger and worry, and can be grateful for everything. Why is compassion the most important element when working in a hospital? Because it is only through a compassionate mind/heart that we start to see everybody as equal, and therefore we start to feel safe and secure ourselves. This in turn makes us a more grounded and flexible practitioner. Real compassion is when we see there is no giver, no gift, and no receiver. This is the state of mind when the most energy flows between you and your client. Whether you are together in a busy hospital or a beautiful spa, compassion can help both you and your client shine more brightly.

The power of compassion can totally transform both ourselves
and others so that our lives become radiant and light.
– Tarthang Tulku, *Openness Mind*

Chapter 35

Reiki Practitioner Burnout in Hospitals

Many Reiki practitioners now are performing hands-on healing in hospitals and hospices all over the world. It is wonderful for practitioners, patients and families to experience the benefits of this element of hands-on healing. However, I often see that after a while of doing these sessions, practitioners start to show symptoms of burnout. These symptoms can range from feeling depleted, worried, or fearful, to physical symptoms like fatigue or headaches, just to name a few.

This mainly happens if the practitioner is feeling too empathic with a client. Empathy means that we sense and feel what the other person is experiencing; going beyond sympathy, we empathize with them. This can trigger empathy distress, where the practitioner becomes overwhelmed by what their client is going through. Often this overwhelming sensation will lead to burnout.

> Too many workers in medical settings suffer from empathy distress which leads to emotional exhaustion.
> – Eve Ekman, Post-Doctoral Scholar at UCSF's Osher Center for Integrative Medicine

The system of Reiki gives us a wonderful tool to combat practitioner burnout; it is one of the precepts.

Do not anger
Do not worry
Be grateful
Practice diligently
Show compassion to yourself and others

The precept/tool to help combat practitioner burnout is compassion.

Compassion is very different from empathy; with compassion, we want to alleviate the client's suffering, but with empathy, we are suffering along with them.

Compassion is where we want to see the client as whole again. This doesn't necessarily mean cured but whole in their mind/heart, which in turn creates an internal happiness for our client. We cannot always cure physical issues; in fact "we" are not "curing" anything. However, we can facilitate within our client a wholesome state of mind/heart. And if they have a wholesome state of mind/heart, they will look at their physical issues from a very different perspective, thus making these issues easier to deal with. This wholesome compassionate state of mind/heart also will help the client and loved ones if the client is passing away. However, if we empathize with our client and she is passing away, we might start to go into empathy distress again.

Lack of empathy certainly doesn't mean that we don't care about our client or her family. But focusing on compassion rather than empathy means that we care about ourselves too, that we care about tending to the state of our own mind/heart. And the clearer, more open, more wholesome our state of mind/heart is, the more we can help to extend this to our client without becoming overwhelmed or burned out.

Compassion creates an expanded spacious mind/heart in which we can witness our clients' suffering without suffering along with them. Instead we start to feel compassion filled with healthy, free-flowing energy which can alleviate their suffering, helping it to dissolve into a wholesome state of mind/heart.

Modern science also shows that compassion is a great antidote to burnout. Research at the University of North Carolina showed that compassion softened depression and stimulated people's moods. The same results were seen in research at Atlanta, Georgia's Emory University, which also showed that practicing compassion reduced subjects' stress levels. Neuroscientist Tania Singer's research shows that compassion protects against empathy distress and enhances energy instead of encouraging burnout.

> The more we care for the happiness of others, the greater our own sense of well-being becomes. Cultivating a close, warm-hearted feeling for others automatically puts the mind at ease. This helps remove whatever fears or insecurities we may have and gives us the strength to cope with any obstacles we encounter.
> – Dalai Lama

Therefore, to combat practitioner burnout, focus on compassion instead of empathy. This of course is not always that easy and this is why within the system of Reiki there are many tools to help us lay bare our innate compassion. Consistently using these tools – meditation practices and techniques, meditating on the precepts, meditating on the mantras and symbols, and practicing Reiju – will help us to build upon all that already is within us, expanding our mind/heart while still feeling grounded and calm. In this way, we can share the benefits of hands-on healing with people in hospitals and hospices without overwhelm and burnout, but instead with compassion and light.

Part 4

Symbols and Mantras

Chapter 36

The Magical Essence of the Symbols

The essence of the symbols is so simple that we could express it in one or two sentences, so simple that we often overlook it. We get carried away with all sorts of interpretations, like that the symbols are magic tools which all by themselves have energy like a magic sword.

There is a wonderful Japanese tale about a sword master who heard about a Tengu – a mythical creature who resided in a deep remote valley and who had a magic sword. The sword master took the long journey to find the Tengu and one day he found her sitting on a log in the forest with her magic sword by her side. The sword master said, "Please can I have your magic sword?" The Tengu replied, "I give you a technique to practice – practice it for 5 years and then you can have my magic sword. But you have to practice every day, if you don't practice every day you do not get it!" The sword master went back home and for 5 years diligently practiced the technique the Tengu had shown him.

After 5 years the sword master made his way back to the remote valley and its mysterious forest. The Tengu was waiting for him, and she said, "I can see you diligently have been practicing for 5 years the technique I showed you; here is my magic sword." However, rather than rushing forward to accept the sword with glee and gratitude, the sword master simply replied, "Thank you, Tengu, but I do not need your magic sword anymore as I have realized that the real magic is inside of me." The Tengu smiled and with one puff disappeared.

The magical essence of the symbols is that they are tools to focus our mind upon, to reawaken a specific inner quality of our own true self. These qualities always have been inside of us; all the symbol does is to call them forth so that we can embody them day and night.

Now of course you may ask, what are these qualities? Again it is very simple. Like the essence of the symbols which can be expressed in two sentences, you can express these qualities in two words – compassion and wisdom

The more we practice with the symbols, the more we find over time that we can embody qualities like compassion and wisdom without even thinking about it. As they become even more a part of our human selves, we no longer need to focus on our tools. Our own magical essence – our true self – will provide all the focus we need.

Chapter 37

Symbols and Mantras the Japanese Way

Many symbols and mantras are used within traditional Japanese spiritual teachings. By looking at these traditional Japanese spiritual practices, we can start to see how Mikao Usui used the symbols and mantras in his teachings.

Within the teachings, the symbols are focus tools; they help us to stay mindful. Now we can ask ourselves, "Mindful of what?" Mindful of not being distracted by the past, present, and future. Because if our mind is distracted by the past, present, and future, our energy also is distracted. And therefore, as energy follows the mind, our hands-on healing sessions also will be distracted.

The symbols, in a way, do not have a power of their own. They are like a sword. A sword doesn't have power on its own either. Sit in a chair and lay a sword in front of you; does it have power? Is it going to rise by itself and slash about? Of course not. What makes the sword powerful? The sword becomes powerful only when we pick it up and handle it. But we have to know how to handle it or else we might cut ourselves. Hence the power really comes from the mind of the person who is handling the sword. This is the same as with the symbols within the system of Reiki. We have to understand in our mind how to handle the symbols and what their real meaning is; that is what will create the power.

The symbols are tools to help us to rediscover our own hidden inner light, our Reiki, our true self. This is why these symbols are taught in Okuden Level II. Okuden means hidden or inner teachings; the symbols and mantras are tools to help us find what is hidden deep inside of us, our true self. To remember what is hidden inside of us, we have to use the symbols and mantras over and over again – on a daily basis and not just once in a while. By meditating on the symbols again and again and again, we start to slowly peel away our layers of ignorance, our anger and worry; this in turn will lay bare our hidden inner great bright light. If we only use the symbols sparingly, then we will never be able to let go of ignorance that is ingrained in our mind, body, and energy, ignorance that covers up our light.

This is also why the symbols and mantras were tools for meditation, meant to help us go within. However, over time they have become very externalized and now often are used only during hands-on healing sessions. By externalizing them, we will find it much harder to see what is hidden inside of our self. Thus, traditionally the symbols are visualized within the mind. Beginning students might draw them with their hands, still seeing them as external tools. But over time, students need to internalize them, to embody the symbols within their own minds.

The symbols also have mantras associated with them. Of the first two symbols within the system of Reiki the mantras are not the name of the symbol; the symbol and mantra are two separate elements. One, the symbol, is a visual aid, and the other, the mantra, is an auditory aid for remembering our true self. We visualize the symbol and repeat the mantra again and again and again. This is a common custom in traditional Japanese spiritual teachings.

For example, in the traditional Japanese spiritual practice of Ajikan, you sit in front of a scroll which has the Sanskrit symbol A (see picture on the front cover) on it. On a historical note, the second symbol within Okuden Reiki II is also derived from a Sanskrit symbol, the kiriku – hrih. During the practice, you rest your mind on this A symbol and start to internalize it so that you become the symbol. At the same time you recite the A sound again and again and again; you do this for up to 45 minutes per session.

Mikao Usui intended the symbols and mantras to be used in his teachings in the same way, especially as he was teaching a spiritual practice. We cannot realize our great bright light if we only use the symbols and mantras once in a while in an external way. We have to internalize them, and we can only do this by meditating on them for a prolonged period of time.

When we practice Mikao Usui's teachings as a spiritual path, as the precepts point out, we need to learn how to meditate upon the symbols and mantras just like the traditional Japanese teachings point out. The more we do this, the more we can let go of our anger and worry, the more grateful and true to our way and our true self we will be, and the more compassionate we will be to ourselves and others.

By embodying the symbols and mantras, we are embodying the precepts. This in turn will free up stuck energy within our body, so that it will start to flow more and more freely, which in turn will make us a clearer vehicle for helping other people. Hence, because our energy is flowing freely, our hands-on healing sessions will happen in a much deeper state, a state of clarity, consciousness, and compassion.

Chapter 38

The Hidden Meaning of the First Symbol

In 2016, as part of my 3-week training in Japan, I spent 5 days on Mt. Omine, which has been a training ground for Shugendo for 1,300 years.

The main temple, Ominesanji, is at the top of the mountain, 1720 meters high. As I stood in front of the temple, I noticed a pillar with a kanji on it and thought, "It looks very similar to the first symbol taught within the system of Reiki." I was intrigued.

I went inside the temple and asked the head priest, Kyosei Yamauchi Sensei, if I could ask him some questions. I drew the first symbol on a piece of paper and as soon as I had finished he said, "This means: go to kami – go to your essence. Go to your essence." This of course means, "Remember your true self."

He explained further that this is an old way of pointing out the metamorphosis, in our current body/form, from being a confused human being to realizing that we are "kami."

Realizing that we are kami is about rediscovering our true self.

He explained that what I had drawn is based on the sosho (cursive) and gyosho (semi-cursive) way of writing the kanji kami 神.

This of course makes perfect sense, as the associated mantra for this symbol is choku rei 直霊, which literally means direct spirit, which in turn is nothing other than our divine spirit – our true self. Both the mantra and the symbol are pointing out the same thing: the metamorphosis to our true self, kami, in this current body.

In the modern system of Reiki, the symbol is often called choku rei, but from a traditional Japanese viewpoint this is not the case. This is why in the teachings of the International House of Reiki, we simply call it Symbol 1. Choku rei is the mantra and the symbol is the visual aspect: two different tools which help us to do the same thing.

But now we come to the important part of this symbol. In modern teachings, this symbol is used externally during a hands-on healing session or during a reiju/initiation/attunement for our client or student. However, we can draw and wave the symbol over a person, thinking, "Go to kami, go to your true self," but that doesn't really work! If it were that easy, we could stand on the corner of the street and wave the symbol over everybody and presto!

Everybody would morph into their true self, would have no more anger and worry, and would be compassionate. Lovely to think about, but we all know that this doesn't really happen!

It would be like saying to a person, "Go and eat." We can't make them eat; they can only do this themselves. It's like the saying, "You can take a horse to the water but you can't make her drink."

So how was the symbol used within Mikao Usui's time? It was used internally, as a tool on which to focus our mind. It was drawn again and again and again in a meditation session. In doing this, we would not so easily get distracted by the past, present, and future, so that we could morph into kami, our true self.

This is the real power behind the symbol: our metamorphosis into kami, into our true self. And it is only from this stage on that our hands-on healing session and reiju/initiation/attunement will take a much deeper form. Because how can I help others to morph into kami, into their true self, if I haven't been there myself?

Thus we can see that Mikao Usui's traditional teachings are to be used internally, to help us so that we can morph into a living kami, the embodiment of our true self. Because it is only at that time that we can let go of our anger and worry, that we can be grateful, true to our way and our true self and can live a compassionate life.

Chapter 39

Deeper Insights into Choku Rei 直霊 (Nao Hi)

When we want to know what Mikao Usui had in mind with his teachings, we need to look not only at traditional Japanese teachings as a whole, but also at what other serious Japanese teachers were teaching at the time.

Here I will compare one aspect of Mikao Usui's teachings to the teachings of Masahisa Goi (1916–1980).

The term chokurei 直霊. Choku (直) means "direct" and rei (霊) means "spirit." Chokurei is the light emanating directly from God to the origin of humanity. Chokurei could be translated as "God in the human world," "Direct Spirit," or "Divine Self."
– Masahisa Goi, *God and Man: Guideposts for Spiritual Peace and Awakening*

People who need not to be reborn into the physical world have experienced the awareness that human beings are one with God, and that awareness is manifested through their actions. Since they are unified with their original, divine Self. [The expression used for divine Self is Choku Rei 直霊.]
– Masahisa Goi, *God and Man: Guideposts for Spiritual Peace and Awakening*

There I encountered my own divine spirit Choku Rei [直霊].
– Masahisa Goi, *Living Like the Blue Sky: 5 talks by Masahisa Goi*

Thus, we can see that choku rei (or nao hi) really points to our true self, our essence, our Reiki, our divine self. This is why it was taught in Okuden Reiki Level II. Okuden means inner teaching; we have to look inside of ourselves to find our true self, our divine self. In Mikao Usui's time, choku rei was used as an internal practice; the mantra was an aid to remember one's own true self. If we were practicing the teachings of that time, we would chant the mantra over and over again until one day we laid bare our choku rei, our true self, our divine self. For people who had a difficult time staying focused while chanting the mantra, Mikao Usui added the symbol. Having to focus on both a mantra and a symbol helped the practitioner to become more mindful, to lessen distraction and stay within the internal practice.

However, over time the mantra and symbol became more and more externalized until the internal practice was almost forgotten.

But if we use the mantra and symbol externally, we will have a hard time rediscovering our choku rei, our true self, our divine self.

Using the mantra and symbol on someone else doesn't really make them rediscover their choku rei, their true self. If this was the case, as said before, we could stand on the corner of our street, say the mantra and wave the symbol over each person and presto; they have rediscovered their choku rei, true self, divine self, and they will be in a permanent state of no more anger and worry, while being grateful and compassionate all the time. But we all know that this doesn't really work! Else we would live in a peaceful world already. We can only rediscover our own choku rei, true self, divine self; no one else can do this for us.

Thus, if you really want to remember your choku rei, your true self, your divine self, turn inwards and start chanting the mantra choku rei for prolonged periods at a time. In doing this, as our outer layers of anger and worry start to fall away over time, our choku rei, true self, divine self can shine through.

Chapter 40

Harmony and Reiki

Each and every master, regardless of the era or the place, heard
the call and attained harmony with heaven and earth.
– Morihei Ueshiba, *The Art of Peace*

The Okuden Level II of the system of Reiki teaches symbols and
mantras. In modern teachings, the second symbol and mantra
is called the emotional/mental symbol. However, within the
traditional teachings of Mikao Usui, the characteristic of this
symbol and mantra is harmony.

Harmony is a quality used in all traditional Japanese spiritual
teachings to remind the practitioner to practice harmony within
herself and with the universe.

The master of harmony alone understands life, and he who
lacks it is foolish in spite of all other knowledge that he might
have acquired.
– Hazrat Inayat Khan, *The Mysticism of Sound and Music*

Attaining harmony within yourself and the universe is one of the
key elements within Mikao Usui's teachings. The first step within
Okuden is to meditate for a long period of time, 6 months, 1 year
or 2 years, on the first symbol and mantra to embody the quality of
earth energy. When we have stabilized that within our own being,
we can take the next step and focus on the second symbol and
mantra for a prolonged period of time. Traditionally, the second
symbol and mantra is associated with heavenly energy and is
connected to Amida Buddha. Amida Buddha is often pictured
descending on a cloud from heaven to help all sentient beings.

In many modern teachings the symbols and mantras are

externalized and only used for hands-on healing sessions with others. However, in Mikao Usui's time, these tools were meant to be meditated upon and embodied by the practitioner. We can see this also by looking at the traditional name for Reiki Level II, Okuden. Okuden translates as hidden or inner teachings; this is pointing to our own hidden, inner true self/Reiki. And to rediscover our true self, we need to internalize these tools.

It is the attainment of harmony which is called heaven.
– Hazrat Inayat Khan, *The Mysticism of Sound and Music*

It is only when we are in harmony with heaven and earth energy that we start to achieve glimpses of our true self/Reiki. This is why all the true masters of old pointed this out. The more we are in harmony, the more these glimpses will, in time, bring to light our own light/true self/Reiki.

Chapter 41

The Non-Dual Nature of Hon Sha Ze Sho Nen

Within Okuden Reiki Level II, we learn the symbol/mantra hon sha ze sho nen 本者是正念.

Literally this mantra translates as "My original nature is a correct thought." Or in a direct way we can say it means "I am right mind" or "I am right mindfulness."

The "I am" in this case is not the ego "I" but our true self, our original nature.

When we look into this translation, we can ask ourselves what is this "right" or "correct" thought? To find the answer we need to look into the fundamental essence of our original nature, our true self. The essence of our original nature is non-duality; thus, the thought which comes forth from this state of mind is a non-dual thought.

In his recently published book, *Zen Chants: Thirty-Five Essential Texts with Commentary*, noted Japanese calligrapher and translator of Buddhist texts Kazuaki Tanahashi states that 正 sho represents non-duality. Therefore, we can also translate hon sha ze sho nen 本者是正念 as "my original nature is a non-dual thought," or "I am non-dual thought."

Interestingly, this doesn't point to distance healing at all. In fact it points towards the opposite of distance healing, as distance implies a dualistic state of mind. So we are not doing distance healing; rather, we simply realize our non-dual nature with everything and set our intent in that space while we rest our mind in the brightness of our non-dual state of mind. But that is easier said than done. Therefore, we can only really remember this non-dual state of mind of our original nature – our true self – if we meditate daily on the symbols and mantras. It is through these kinds of meditations that we discover the deeper layers of Mikao Usui's teachings.

All of this makes perfect sense as, first and foremost, the system of Reiki is a spiritual practice. Thus, it helps the practitioner to reach a state of mind of non-duality.

In fact Hon Sha Ze Sho Nen 本者是正念 has a close relation with the Tendai Hongaku teachings 天台本覚思想.

Hongaku is the original state of enlightenment. Hongaku means that everything is enlightened already, everything has a non-dual nature. Or in other words, everything is the great bright light already; we just have forgotten this.

> Komyo (the light [of the Buddha]) emphasizes the notion that there is no place between heaven and earth that Buddha-nature, and therefore original enlightenment, does not permeate.
> – *The Bodymind Experience in Japanese Buddhism: A Phenomenological Perspective of Kukai and Dogen* by David Edward Shaner

Thus, we can say that hon sha ze sho nen is a signpost for helping us to rediscover our own original great bright light of non-duality: our true self.

Mikao Usui pointed this out by teaching some of his serious Shinpiden students the dai kômyô, the Shinpiden Reiki III symbol/mantra.

> Komyo exists in me and I exist in Komyo.
> – Note from a student of Mikao Usui, supplied by Hiroshi Doi.

The more we start to explore Mikao Usui's teachings from a traditional Japanese perspective, rather than a modern Japanese perspective, the more we start to really see what Mikao Usui was trying to teach his students, a deep spiritual practice. And in this practice we can, over time, rediscover our original nature of non-duality.

Chapter 42

The Deeper Layers of "Distance" Healing

Within the system of Reiki there is a practice which is commonly called "distance" healing. Many modern Reiki schools teach that you do this by "sending" something to someone – by using a pillow or stuffed animal, by placing your hand on your leg, by making a bridge, etc...

However, traditionally this was not the case at all. We can see this clearly when we look at Mikao Usui's teachings within Okuden Reiki Level II.

First of all, Okuden means "inner teachings" which means when we do "distance" healing, we need to bring it inwards – inwards into our mind/heart. Using a pillow, making a bridge, using our leg – all of these things make the practice external, "sending" our focus outwards.

Secondly, when we learn "distance" healing we learn the symbol and mantra Hon Sha Ze Sho Nen 本者是正念.

Translated, Hon Sha Ze Sho Nen 本者是正念 means: "my original nature is a non-dual thought." As you can see, it says nothing about "distance" healing. Rather, it states that we need to realize that our original nature is a non-dual thought. Traditionally this was done through extended periods of meditating on the symbol and chanting the mantra.

If we teach our students to use a pillow, a leg, a bridge, or that they are "sending" something, then we keep reinforcing the idea that there is a distance which we need to overcome. But if we really look deeply into the true nature of reality, we will see that there is no distance at all. We are all interconnected.

This is also why when we perform "distance" healing we have to let go of the idea that we need to connect to someone, or an animal, or a tree, as we are already interconnected. The more we instill the idea that we need to connect, the more we teach ourselves that we are not interconnected at all. So better straightaway to teach that we are already connected and that all we need to do is remember that we are interconnected in the first place – no need to connect!

But why do so many people teach that we need to connect and that it is all external? This is because there is a lot of worry and fear involved, which in essence comes from our ego. Think about it; if we realize that we are already interconnected with a friend who has cancer and we are one with the person, then we are also one with the cancer! This concept can trigger a lot of worry and fear for the untrained practitioner. (It also can lead to the idea that we need "protection" in our practice, but that is another topic altogether!) This is why traditionally "distance" healing was taught in the latter part of Okuden. By that time the student had overcome most of their worry and fear already, which is also pointed out within the precepts. Contemplating and meditating with the precepts is a fundamental practice in Shoden Reiki Level I.

Thus by practicing that we are all interconnected when we perform "distance" healing – without the need for a pillow, a leg, a bridge, or sending – the practitioner starts to loosen their worry and fear. This is why traditionally this practice was also for the practitioner, to soften their ego, their grip – attachment – on their small self. In this way, the practitioner can become more open, moving towards and embracing their true self instead of clinging to a small, fearful, worried self.

This is why it is so important to practice the deeper aspects of "distance" healing, so that we can realize our true nature, our inner great bright light in which we realize that we are all interconnected already. This interconnectedness will also help us to become more compassionate to ourselves because we have let go of our own ego and self-cherished concepts; this in turn helps us to becomes more compassionate to others.

So next time when you perform "distance" healing, give your ego a kick in the butt and instead feel the interconnectedness with your friend, with your animal, with their illness. Feel the interconnectedness with all that is and take a step deeper into the spiritual teachings of Mikao Usui.

Part 5

History

Chapter 43

The Different Names of Mikao Usui

In the time of Mikao Usui, it was very common for people to have different names. These might include birth names, artist/style names (goh), popular names, Buddhist names, and/or posthumous names (戒名 kaimyo/imina).

Mikao Usui, founder, practitioner, and teacher of the system of Reiki, also had different names.

First of all, we know him as Mikao Usui 臼井甕男.
His artist/style name (goh) is Akiho/Gyohan 暁帆.
Mikao Usui's posthumous (戒名 kaimyo) name is:

> Reizan-in Shuyo Tenshin Koji 霊山院秀譽天心居士
> 霊 – Rei as in Reiki
> 山 – Zan (as in mountain)
> 院 – In (a ranking/title of deceased)
> 秀 – Shu (preeminent)
> 譽 – Yo (given to one who has completed the Fivefold Transmission in Pure Land Sect)
> 天 心 – Tenshin (zenith, divine will)
> 居 士 – Koji (given to lay Buddhists)

I think his kaimyo (戒名) 霊山院秀譽天心居士 is worthy of his [Mikao Usui's] achievements. As you know, 霊山 means the sacred mountain, which is the mother of Reiki as well as Japanese Religion.
– Takeda Hakusai Ajari

It was also very common in Mikao Usui's time to take on the family name and one's father's name after the father's death. This is why it is said that Mikao Usui also was known by these names:

No-Tsunetane: (之) 常胤

No-Uzaemon: (之) 宇左衛門

Judith Rabinovitch, Professor Emerita of Japanese Language and Culture at the University of Montana explains:

> Sometimes, even in modern times, in the case of old, traditional families, the eldest son (or the eldest surviving son) will take his father's name upon the latter's death. It would therefore not be exceptional for Mikao Usui to have used his own father's name. Regarding the insertion of "No" in front of the above names, Tsunetane and Uzaemon: as in Usui/Chiba no Uzaemon or Chiba no Tsunetane: in premodern times, but especially the court period, family names were written first, followed by the grammatical particle No (a sort of nominal linker and sometimes like an apostrophe "s" in English). Therefore, the great poet of the court was referred to as Fujiwara No Teika, rather than Fujiwara Teika in his day. (Teika "of" the Fujiwara family.) This is not part of the name itself but rather a grammatical linkage between surname and the given name that followed. In modern times, this linkage no longer is made.

As you can see, when doing research into Mikao Usui, we need to look at all the different names he was known by. Just as it is when practicing, when researching the system of Reiki, there always is something new to learn.

And also in teaching the system of Reiki, there always is something new to learn! Each student, each class is unique, and at any given moment in time, students and teachers are at a different point along in their practice, their experiences, and their healing journey. This means that we all can learn from one another. So let's embrace each moment of this journey where, by any other name, student is teacher and teacher is student.

Chapter 44

The Esoteric Teachings of Mikao Usui

Within the precepts we can find this phrase:

招福の祕法
shou fuku no hi hou
pronounced: show fuku no hehoo
invite blessings of secret method

This is commonly translated as "the secret method to invite blessings." But 祕法 hihou or hiho also can be translated as "esoteric teachings." Hi 祕 means secret, hidden, esoteric, spiritual, and deeper.

Hou 法 means Dharma, reality, true principle, method, teachings, and original nature.

Therefore, by using this phrase in the introduction to his five precepts, Mikao Usui was pointing out his esoteric teachings. But many people get confused by the word esoteric.

A leaflet handed out at Mt. Koyasan, the main temple complex of the Shingon tradition in Japan, explains what esoteric means in a very simple and clear way: the word "esoteric" is used within Shingon Buddhism to indicate two teachings. First, that the Buddhas preach by adjusting their teachings according to the ability of their audiences to comprehend, and so to reserve some teachings until beings are ready for them. In this case, the Buddha wisely holds back teachings temporarily until the listener is ready for them... Esoteric here does not mean a willful withholding of the teachings to a select few. The teachings of Shingon Esoteric Buddhism are available to anyone, but require careful sequential preparation through several stages. The word "esoteric" is used to emphasize the need to train ourselves to realize what was there all along but what was hidden to us by our own ignorance. We can see very clearly within Mikao Usui's teachings that he also was teaching according to his students' spiritual development. Some of his students weren't ready for the next stage of his teachings. We can see this very clearly if, for example, we look at the Reiki III Shinpiden symbol/mantra dai kômyô. Some of Mikao Usui's students were taught this symbol/mantra and yet others were not.

Reiki researcher and teacher Hiroshi Doi explains: "Usui Sensei called Shinpiden students into his room one by one, saying, 'You have been working on developing your pipe of Reiki since you had it opened until you learned Okuden Koki. But that is not enough, as you were chosen to be a Shinpiden practitioner. From now on you must devote yourself to give the Light to as many people as possible.' And he showed a piece of paper with three Kanji characters of Dai, Ko and Myo on it, which indicated the basic consciousness of Shinpiden practitioner." Hiroshi Doi got this information, and more, from an Aikido Shihan whose grandfather was a student of Mikao Usui.

When we look at the whole system of Reiki, we also can see that Mikao Usui was teaching the esoteric way, depending on the spiritual development of his students. He was teaching some of his students just a very basic form of hands-on healing and yet others he was teaching a very deep spiritual practice, with meditations to lay bare what has always been there: Reiki – our true self.

Usui Sensei had no standard curriculum, and the length of time of the training depended on the spiritual progress of each student. It is said that he gave one-on-one lectures mainly on the right mental attitude needed for spiritual advancement based on his own experience.
– Hiroshi Doi

In his teachings, Mikao Usui also was encouraging learning

in stages. Shoden was the beginner level and it is said that he had only around 2,000 students. Okuden was the next stage; for this level, he had only about 80 or so students. Hence we can start to see that students had to prepare for the next level and if they weren't ready, he did not teach them. The next stage was Shinpiden and Mikao Usui had only about 22 or so students for this level. But that doesn't mean that all his students at this level were taught the same; again, he was teaching according to their spiritual development. This means that some of his Shinpiden students only knew the hands-on healing parts while others were offered the deeper teachings. Again, this is why some of his Shinpiden level students were taught the dai kômyô and others not.

> Usui Sensei personally selected from among qualified Okuden Koki level students those who possessed a high level of spirituality, and offered them further instructions at Shinpiden level. Shinpiden students were selected to receive Usui Sensei's direct private teachings and learn how to aim for Anshin Ritsumei.
> – Hiroshi Doi

To again quote the Shingon leaflet, "The word 'esoteric' is used to emphasize the need to train ourselves to realize what was there all along but what was hidden to us by our own ignorance." The deepest aim of Mikao Usui's teachings was to help his students to remember their true self – Reiki, that which was there all along in all of us but was hidden by our own anger and worry, by not being grateful and true to our way and our being, and by not being compassionate to ourselves and others. The true self often is hidden by our ignorance. But it was not a matter of Mikao Usui simply giving each student a magic key to unlock the door to the true self. Rather than just being taught information or being shown a particular practice, the student had to be ready to take the teachings into their own hands and practice the meditation practices. With continuing teachings, practice and direct experience, each in its own time, the student could realize this true self within themselves.

Chapter 45

The Roots of the System of Reiki

Without the roots a plant will not grow and bear fruit.

To really understand the system of Reiki, we need to go back to the roots that Mikao Usui planted for his teachings. By exploring and practicing the roots, we can pick the real fruits of the system of Reiki.

Many teachers look for these roots within Mrs. Takata's or Chujiro Hayashi's teachings. However, due to extensive research we now know that both of these teachers changed Mikao Usui's teachings. Therefore we cannot find the real roots there.

Some people may not be happy with this section as they have invested much into their system, but I think we need to be truthful and honest when we talk about Mikao Usui's teachings. Changes happen, but let's be open and upfront about them. Here we examine a few of these changes.

Changes to the system by the Usui Reiki Ryoho Gakkai

The Usui Reiki Ryoho Gakkai is a very elusive group of teachers and practitioners in Japan. Over the years some members have taught publicly to outsiders and informed them of some of their teachings. In 2001, we met with a Gakkai member in Tokyo who explained some of their teachings.

Both this person and Hiroshi Doi, another well-known Gakkai member, state that even within the Gakkai the teachings changed after Mikao Usui's death.

> Dento Reiki [Usui Reiki Ryoho Gakkai] as it was practiced by members of the Usui Reiki Ryoho Gakkai before Usui sensei's death drastically changed after his passing and even more after

the end of World War II.

– Hiroshi Doi, *A Modern Reiki Method for Healing*

Thus to know the roots of Mikao Usui's teachings we cannot completely rely on the Usui Reiki Ryoho Gakkai; we need to dig deeper to Mikao Usui himself.

Changes to the system by Chujiro Hayashi

Like many other Japanese and non-Japanese Reiki researchers, Hiroshi Doi also rediscovered numerous changes made by Chujiro Hayashi.

This is what we now know Hayashi changed...Taken from an interview with Hiroshi Doi in the *Reiki News Magazine*:

William Rand: How did Dr. Hayashi's style of Reiki change after he left the Gakkai?

Doi Sensei: It is not that his style changed when he left the Gakkai, but that a new style was developed from the beginning of his Kenkyu Kai. A recipient, except a seriously ill person, was to sit when receiving treatment; this sitting position was changed to a lying position on a table. The treatment method was changed from one-on-one to several-on-one... An original hands-on position was developed and the new Reiki Ryoho Shinshin or "Guidelines for Reiki Healing Method" were created. A new system of conferring and passing [reiju/initiation/attunement] on Reiki Ryoho was established, and a monthly five-day workshop was held at which Okuden was given. While at the Gakkai, the navel and the Tanden were considered important, the energy centers like the meridian lines of acupuncture, Tsubo, or vital points, and chakras, etc. became important.

Hiroshi Doi explains this even further in his book *Modern Reiki Method for Healing*, and in his manuals:

But I could find signs that he [Chujiro Hayashi] had already converted the "Usui method" into the "Hayashi method" even before he taught Takata Sensei. He seemed to try modernizing Reiki-ho based on his medical knowledge and experience as a practical therapist. Next, although Hayashi Sensei advertised to the public that he taught "Usui" Reiki Ryoho after he had become independent of the Gakkai, he actually taught "Hayashi" Reiki. He adopted his own theories and techniques aimed at curing disease.

The basic 12 hand positions and the attunements procedures [with the symbols and mantras] we use today are all derived from Hayashi-sensei's techniques.

Reiju, as currently practiced, is said to be based upon the form developed by Hayashi-sensei, and then given to Hawayo Takata.

Thus we can see that Hayashi changed many aspects of the system of Reiki. Therefore to know the roots and eat the real fruit of the system of Reiki, we also cannot look completely at Hayashi's teachings.

Changes to the system by Mrs. Takata

Even though Mrs. Takata followed Hayashi's teachings, she knew of the real roots of the system of Reiki; yet she didn't incorporate these within her teachings. We can see this from recordings of Mrs. Takata from her student John Harvey Gray:

When John studied with Takata, he made over 20 audio tapes of her lectures and classes. On one of the tapes she discusses travelling to Japan in order to teach her approach to Reiki. While there, she met some Japanese citizens who were actively practicing and preserving Reiki as they understood it in

Japan. Takata regarded their approach as entirely valid, but inappropriate for the West. It was highly complex, required years of training and was closely intertwined with religious practices. She felt these factors would deter students in the West and hobble the spread of Reiki through the world at a time when, in her view, it was urgently needed.
– *Hand to Hand* by John Harvey Gray

Here we can see that what Mrs. Takata was teaching was not what teachers in Japan, who were "actively practicing and preserving" Mikao Usui's teachings, were practicing. These also were intertwined with religious practices – practices from Buddhism, teachings like Tendai and Shugendo for example – which Mrs. Takata chose to omit from her teachings in the West.

So again, to rediscover the roots of the system of Reiki and the fruit Mikao Usui wanted us to eat, we also cannot look completely at Mrs. Takata's teachings.

This is one of the reasons I study with Japanese Shingon, Tendai, and Shugendo priests, so that I can gain a clearer understanding of what Mrs. Takata already was pointing out about Mikao Usui's teachings. This in turn will help me to teach the roots of Usui Reiki Ryoho to our students.

Usui Reiki Ryoho, what is in a name?

Mikao Usui originally called his system Usui Reiki Ryoho; we can see this written within the precepts.

Reiki stands for "true self," Ryo stands for "to heal," and Ho stands for "teaching, method or Dharma." Thus Usui Reiki Ryoho means Usui's teachings to heal one's true self. Or in other words: "Usui's teachings to rediscover our true self."

It doesn't mean a hands-on healing method; rather it is a method to rediscover our true self, from which we can practice hands-on healing. Therefore, real hands-on healing is a product of rediscovering our true self. The spiritual level of the practitioner directly reflects the effect of Reiki. In a sense, the more you are enlightened, the more the effectiveness of Reiki enhances. The more you practice Reiki for saving others, the brighter your innate light shines to drive away clouds covering your mind. I think this is the quintessence of Reiki.

– Takeda Hakusai Ajari

Traditionally in Japan you would change the name of the teachings, Usui Reiki Ryoho, to a different name only if you changed the system. If you didn't change the system you would keep the same name, Usui Reiki Ryoho, because this showed that your teachings flowed from the source of the founder – showing respect to the founder.

Thus we also can see that both Hayashi and Mrs. Takata changed their teachings because they both changed the name of their style of teaching. Hayashi changed his name to "Hayashi Reiki Ryoho Kenkyukai." Some who teach in the lineage of Hayashi have changed the name again, indicating that they also have changed Hayashi's teachings. If they hadn't, why change the name of the teachings? Japanese have a very deep respect for teachings and therefore only would change the name if they felt they had changed the teachings. To do otherwise wouldn't be respectful to the founder of the system.

Mrs. Takata, even though in some occasions she called it Usui Reiki Ryoho, felt the need to change it to Usui Shiki Ryoho.

The Roots

So, with so many teachers having changed the system of Reiki, how do we find its roots? We can find the root of Mikao Usui's teachings by meditating on the tools he left us.

I've used this analogy before, but it bears repeating: say you want to know everything about a tree. You could buy a book about trees and read it. Now you think, "I know everything about a tree!" But do you really? No; you know the author's idea about what a tree is, based on his/her research, knowledge, experience, thoughts. This is the same when you go to a class – you hear the teacher's ideas.

We could cut down the tree and put it under the microscope and investigate it all intellectually. But that still doesn't help us to know really what a tree is! In the same way, after you go to a class, you could read your manual and notes over and over, to try to better understand or to memorize the ideas and teachings you heard about.

Do either of these methods help you to know what a tree is, or to know the teachings of the system of Reiki? Or does direct experience help you more?

The best option would be to become One with the tree; now we know what it means to be a tree.

The best option would be, as Mikao Usui said in the precepts, to "practice diligently" his teachings.

But that is not as easy as reading a book or going to a class or knowing it intellectually. It is hard practice and it takes time.

We know also that Mikao Usui created his system after he sat meditating on a mountaintop for 21 days! To be able to do this 21-day practice, you first need to have practiced the 3-day and then the 7-day practices, building up gradually so that your mind/body/energy are better able to deal with it. And before you can do a 3- or 7-day practice, you need to have been practicing for a long, long time. This also is what Mrs. Takata pointed out in the quote from *Hand to Hand*; it was a practice which was highly complex, required years and years of training and was intertwined with religious practices.

What if you meditated for 20 minutes every day on the first symbol and mantra? What if you meditated for 20 minutes every day on the precepts? What if you practiced the meditation practice jōshin kokyū hō 20 minutes every day? This might take years and years but only then can we truly rediscover what Mikao Usui left us.

> Though his [Mikao Usui] one-on-one Shinpiden lecture did not include healing training, I also heard that Usui Sensei's mentorship greatly enhanced the healing ability of many of the Shinpiden practitioners, as it strengthened their resonance with the Universe and encouraged the awareness that a human is the small universe derived from the Great Universe.
> – Interview with Hiroshi Doi in *Reiki News Magazine*

Why did Mikao Usui's Shinpiden training not include healing training? Because he knew from his own experience that the real healing came from the unification with the universe and this was what he was teaching his Shinpiden students. And we all know that if we have direct experiences of this unification, that this will greatly enhance our healing ability.

The Fruit

Thus if we say we practice the system of Reiki according to Mikao Usui, we also want to know what the fruit is of Mikao Usui's teachings, not the fruit of Chujiro Hayashi's or Mrs. Takata's teachings.

This is not to say that Hayashi's teachings are not valid or that Mrs. Takata's teachings are not correct. Both are valid in their own right; but because they both changed so much of the system, they are not the roots of the system of Reiki. Therefore the fruit will be Hayashi's fruit or Mrs. Takata's fruit, not Mikao Usui's.

To get the idea in our mind of the fruit of Mikao Usui, we need to go back to the roots of his teachings, the real essence.

Traditionally in Mikao Usui's time, Reiki meant your true self, your innate great bright light. Therefore the fruit of the system of Reiki is the rediscovering of our true self, the embodiment of the precepts. This is what in Japan is called Satori or Anshin Ritsumei.

So the old Gakkai members said that Usui Sensei taught the way to Satori very intensely to those who had achieved a certain level.
– *A Modern Reiki Method for Healing* by Hiroshi Doi

This fruit is symbolized by a symbol/mantra which Mikao Usui put in his system in Shinpiden Reiki Level III – dai kômyô.

Dai kômyô means great bright light, it is the light of our true self.

Usui Sensei called Shinpiden students into his room one by one, saying, "You have been working on developing your pipe of Reiki since you had it opened until you learned Okuden Koki. But that is not enough, as you were chosen to be a Shinpiden practitioner. From now on you must devote yourself to give the Light to as many people as possible." And he showed a piece of paper with three Kanji characters of Dai, Ko and Myo on it, which indicated the basic consciousness of Shinpiden practitioner.
– Hiroshi Doi got this information, and more, from an Aikido Shihan whose grandfather was a student of Mikao Usui.

So dig deep in your practice, go deeper than Hayashi's teachings and Mrs. Takata's teachings. Go all the way down to the roots of Mikao Usui and you will start to rediscover a whole new treasure trove of teachings and experiences; you will start to rediscover your true self. And there you will find the sweetest fruit of all.

Chapter 46

Rediscovering Our Original Nature

There are many practices within the system of Reiki, but Mikao Usui pointed out again and again that the essential focus is rediscovering our original nature. This is because it is only through this rediscovery that we can help others heal with compassion and wisdom.

In the *Reiki Ryoho Hikkei*, a manual handed out by the Usui Reiki Ryoho Gakkai in Japan, it states that Mikao Usui said, "If you can't heal yourself how can you heal others?"

A very clear and direct instruction pointing towards this essential focus is one of the Okuden Reiki II symbols/mantras hon sha ze sho nen 本者是正念. This symbol/mantra is commonly used to do distance healing but in Mikao Usui's time this was not the case; it was a tool to rediscover our own original nature.

Recently I had a conversation with a Japanese Tendai priest in Japan and he said that for him 本者是正念 hon sha ze sho nen has a close relationship with the Tendai Hongaku teachings 天台本覚思想.

Hongaku is the original state of enlightenment. Hongaku means that everything is originally enlightened already, or in other words that everything is the great bright light already, we just have forgotten.

Hon sha ze sho nen 本者是正念 translates as, "My original nature is a correct thought."

What is this correct thought? Is it the thought that we can do distance healing? No, of course not. This thought points straight towards our original nature. It is the thought that we are originally the great bright light already.

This is also pointed out within the Shinpiden Reiki III symbol/ mantra dai kômyô.

Komyo (the light [of the Buddha]) emphasizes the notion that there is no place between heaven and earth that Buddha-nature, and therefore original enlightenment, does not permeate.
–*The Bodymind Experience in Japanese Buddhism: A Phenomenological Perspective of Kukai and Dogen* by David Edward Shaner

Thus both hon sha ze sho nen and dai kômyô are doing the same thing: pointing towards our original nature.

Komyo exists in me and I exist in Komyo.
– Note from a student of Mikao Usui, supplied by Hiroshi Doi

The precepts point to the rediscovery of our original nature out as well. Because it is only in the state of our original nature, our great bright light, that we have no more anger and worry, that we are honest, humble, and compassionate.

But why did he feel the need to remind us in so many ways about our original nature?

Because he realized that we must first heal ourselves before we can heal others.

This leads us to the question of what Mikao Usui thought healing was. We can find the answer in his teachings. Our original nature is also the deepest state of healing. This can also be seen within the precepts, because the precepts do not discuss physical issues at all, but rather state of mind. If we are rediscovering our own original nature we can help others to rediscover theirs.

Therefore the essential focus of the system of Reiki is foremost about rediscovering our original nature. But how do we do this?

Hongaku – original enlightenment is explained in the Jimon Tendai text of Hongaku-zan in a symbolic way as "beans." Everything has original enlightened beans within it, all we have to do is water them, give them light and keep the weeds out.

Within the system of Reiki the rain, the sun, and the weeding is done through meditating on the precepts, meditating on the symbols and mantras, practicing the meditations like jōshin kokyū hō and being in a meditative state of mind during reiju/initiation/attunement.

Chapter 47

Does History Help Us to Embody the Precepts?

> History is not the soil of happiness. The periods of happiness are blank pages in it.
> – Georg Wilhelm Friedrich Hegel

Often I am asked if I teach a lot about the history of Mikao Usui and his teachings in our classes.

For me the most important element within Mikao Usui's teachings is to embody the precepts in our daily life:

Do not anger
Do not worry
Be grateful
Be true to your way and your true self
Be compassionate to yourself and others

Teaching a lot about the history of the system of Reiki doesn't necessarily help us to embody the precepts. It might give us some kind of framework or platform, but that is about it.

> The past is malleable and flexible, changing as our recollection interprets and re-explains what has happened.
> – Peter L. Berger

For me, to embody the precepts we need to learn and practice in class the meditation practices, the symbols and mantras, hands-on healing – elements that I see as more integral to the system of Reiki than its history. Through this actual practice, the teacher can then guide the students. The teacher sees how the students are practicing and thus can adjust the practice accordingly.

For example, a yoga teacher would not necessarily spend a lot of time in class on the history of yoga either. Rather, she would teach the practice and have the students do it. This is the same when we go to a Tai Chi class; we start to practice the methods because it is only through the methods and not through the history that we start to embody the teachings.

In essence, it also doesn't matter so much who, what and where Mikao Usui taught. What matters most is that we facilitate a change within ourselves and our students so that we become less angry and worried, so we become more grateful and true to our way and our true self, and so we become more compassionate to ourselves and others.

Plus, if we focus too much on the history and we state as a teacher that this history is the true and correct one, then we are in fact creating a possibility for more anger and worry! Because now we could get angry and worried if someone speaks about and teaches a different viewpoint of the history.

> History is the version of past events that people have decided to agree upon.
> – Napoleon Bonaparte

Therefore, rather than focusing on the history, I spend more time discussing the practices so that the student understands why they are taught. And we spend time actually practicing the practices so that the student gains a direct experience and is inspired to continue and deepen the practice.

Chapter 48

Comparing Mikao Usui's Teachings with Seishin Kenkyu Kai

Seishin Kenkyu Kai was started by Kuwabara Toshiro (1873–1906). According to Christopher Harding, in *Religion and Psychotherapy in Modern Japan*, Seishin Kenkyu Kai was centered around four concepts:

1 – Mind is energy, a moving agent inherent in everything. Everything, living or not, has a mind.
2 – Each mind can affect other minds.
3 – This understanding of mind can be applied to the universe.
4 – If we stop worrying and become free from all distracting thoughts, the stable mind will appear in us. This stable mind is an offshoot of the great mind of the universe. When we enter this state we can work wonders.

In these four principles, we can see many similarities with Mikao Usui's teachings.

1 – Mind is energy.

This is the same as what Mikao Usui taught. There is a note from a student of Mikao Usui which says, "Everything in the Universe possesses Reiki without any exception." We can see that in essence, Reiki means true self means pure mind.

2 – Each mind can affect other minds.

Hon sha ze sho nen is about Right Mind, or a state of oneness. In this way we see that Usui was showing how each mind can affect other minds.

3 – This understanding of mind can be applied to the universe.

Another note from a student of Mikao Usui states, "We humans hold the Great Reiki that fills the Great Universe." We can see that Usui was teaching that we affect the universe, and the universe affects us.

4 – If we stop worrying and become free from all distracting thoughts, the stable mind will appear in us. This stable mind is an offshoot of the great mind of the universe. When we enter this state we can work wonders.

One of the Reiki precepts is "do not worry." In fact, all of the precepts are about the mind. From this we can see that Usui was reminding us that it is our unstable mind which separates us from our true self. When we are aligned with our true self, we can access our inner ability to heal.

Some Japanese Reiki researchers say that Mikao Usui took his precepts from a book written by Bizan Suzuki in 1914 but I personally do not believe this. The concepts of the precepts were very common at that time, especially around the late 1800s/early 1900s. As we can see, Toshiro-san also used the concept of worry in his teachings, and he died in 1906! The concepts of gyō, compassion, and anger were also very common concepts much earlier than 1914. At this time in Japan there were many people starting to open up old esoteric teachings and they all shared common threads. We can imagine Mikao Usui weaving many threads of thought together to bring us the system of Reiki that we practice today.

Part 6

Teaching

Chapter 49

How to Find the Right Teacher

Many people often ask me how to find the right teacher. It is a difficult question as we all feel attracted to different teachers and different teaching styles.

However, if looking for a teacher myself I would look at one very important aspect: his/her direct experience. The more the teacher has had a direct experience of what they are teaching, the deeper their inner wisdom and compassion is and the more direct their teachings are.

Direct experience = deeper inner wisdom and compassion = more direct teaching. Say I am looking for a teacher to guide me into remembering my inner great bright light, my true self.

Would I go for a teacher who has never had a direct experience of this and yet teaches meditations and practices to remember this great bright light?

Would I go for a teacher who had one experience and because of this thinks he knows it all and therefore doesn't feel the need for further practices?

Or would I go to a teacher who has had multiple experiences of her inner great bright light and who keeps practicing so that she can be in that space more and more?

I would go to the latter one because that teacher has had numerous direct experiences and is dedicated to continuing exploring and practicing.

Many direct experiences + continued practice = deeper connection to true self.

Picking the first teacher would be like asking a guide to help us to climb to the top of a mountain when the guide has never been there. The second guide has been only once to the top of the mountain and thus still can lose his way. But the third one has explored many aspects of the mountain and yet keeps returning to climb it again and again, maybe finding a new perspective here, or a less rocky path there. So she is the best guide of all.

Within the system of Reiki we can ask ourselves the same question. Would you like to train with a teacher who just learned how to do a Reiju but never really did a Shinpiden Reiki III class? Would you like to learn with a teacher who just did a Shinpiden Reiki III class but never really kept practicing the meditations taught within the system? Or would you like to train with a teacher who has done a Shinpiden Reiki III class but keeps exploring and going deeper to remember her true self?

Of course the best teacher would again be the latter one. Why? Because she has been climbing that mountain up and down and up and down and knows many different paths of the mountain.

But this is so hard to find out as we do not know what to look for. We can ask the teacher if he has been to the top of the mountain but he can just make it up. Therefore we might need to work with different teachers until we find the right one to guide us deeper and deeper into remembering our true self. Along the way, it also is most important to continue with our own practice, to expand and deepen our experiences and to cultivate our wisdom and compassion.

One other element is that different people like different paths to the top of the mountain. Some like the steep path, some the zigzag path, some like to walk fast while others slow. Some like to stop along the way while others do not need to rest. The teacher who has explored the mountain again and again and again not only will know all the different paths, but also will have the insight of what different people may need. This means that this kind of teacher is not stuck to one particular method but has become more flexible. This kind of teacher teaches according to the students' spiritual progress and requirements, meeting them where they are on their own individual path. This teacher is the real teacher.

Experts in all the Ways can hardly be called masters if, beyond their various techniques, they have not yet severed themselves from fixation.
– Yagyu Munenori, *The Swordsman's Handbook: Samurai Teachings on the Path of the Sword*

Chapter 50

More Than One Teacher

Many of the students and/or teachers of old had more than one teacher for their spiritual development. This is because different teachers focus on different elements of the teachings. One teacher, for example, might be an expert on chanting mantras, while the other teacher might be an expert on healing rituals.

Some teachers even sent their students to a different teacher for a while to learn a specific method of meditation in which they themselves were not that skilled. This was not seen as an issue at all, but rather a benefit.

Most of the time a student's main teacher was the one who showed the student their true self for the first time. But that didn't mean that the student could not study with different teachers.

However, many modern teachers want their students studying only with them as there seems to be a fear of "contaminating" the teachings. The teachings therefore become very strict and if you become a teacher in that specific method, you can only teach that specific way. Plus, if you mix in a different idea or practice, you will no longer be able to teach that system. That way of teaching is in fact very limited. Teachers are there to help expand students' minds, not to narrow them.

I personally see expanding your learning horizons as a wonderful way of exploring different teachers and different styles. Yes, of course it is good to have one main teacher, but it also is good to explore what others are doing and saying. This will help you as a student to gain a much deeper understanding of the system you are practicing. And it will help you to open your mind.

Plus, if we want to be a teacher and want to practice in an organic way which comes from our own heart, then we need to become more fluid. We need to be able to add certain ideas and practices which we personally feel express the teachings in true ways that will benefit our students. A spiritual teaching is based on compassion and if we want to teach different students according to their spiritual development, we need to be flexible to do so.

If we claim to be teaching a spiritual practice, then as teachers we need to support students in helping them to rediscover their true self, which is the ultimate aim in any kind of spiritual tradition. And we can only do that by setting the student free, free to explore and free to expand their mind. If we put our teachings and the student in a box, we therefore are limiting their spiritual growth. If we remove these box-like boundaries and restrictions, then the students' spiritual growth, like the compassion in setting them free, can be limitless.

Chapter 51

Teaching Others Comes from Our Own Direct Experience

Teaching other people a spiritual practice is a wonderful tool for sharing compassion and wisdom around the world. But how do we teach and where do these teachings come from?

The most important element of teaching a spiritual practice is the teacher's own direct experience of the spiritual practices they are teaching. This direct experience creates openness in their mind/heart through which the energy starts to flow more freely through their being. The more open their mind/heart becomes, the more this openness starts to emanate from their whole being. It might even become so open that the compassionate energy from the teacher's mind/heart emanates throughout the whole meditation room. And this is the space where the real teachings come from.

The student now can entrain, or fall into rhythm with, the compassionate expanded luminous energy that comes from the teacher's own direct experience of their true self. Through this entrainment the students, if they are ready and open, can gain a direct experience of their own true self. This direct experience cannot be expressed intellectually; we cannot point out to someone what is indescribable: their true self. Yet the teacher can facilitate the space in which the student can rediscover this in a direct experience, without words or symbolic language.

However, this can only start to happen if the teacher herself has a direct experience of her own luminous nature. Through dedicated meditation practices over time, the teacher has taken away the lampshades of worry, fear, anger, and attachments and therefore her light emanates all around her.

Facilitating this kind of experience will take the students to a much deeper level than just the intellectual understanding can do.

Intellectually we can understand how to cook a wonderful meal, but it is only after we have the direct experience of cooking and eating it, that it will become real.

If the teacher is just repeating instructions on certain meditation practices which he learned, but only applied basically in his own life without deep and consistent practice, then he is just repeating what he has heard or read. This kind of teaching likely will not facilitate a direct experience of entrainment within the students.

Nowadays many teachers use words like oneness and emptiness, but these are just words. Oneness and emptiness only become alive when the teacher has had numerous direct experiences of this state of oneness and emptiness. Just intellectualizing is not enough; it needs to become a direct experience.

A real spiritual teacher therefore will teach from her own direct experience so that her teachings will become alive with vibrant compassionate luminosity. Teachings like these will help students draw vibrancy, luminosity, wisdom and compassion into their own mind/heart so that they, in turn, can radiate these qualities out to others, and to the world.

Chapter 52

Flexibility in Teaching and Practicing

When your chi is in harmony and tranquil, it will be active and flowing, but it has no fixed form; and without using strength, it will be naturally strong.

– Issai Chozanshi, *The Demon's Sermon on the Martial Arts*

The deeper we go into our personal practice, the more flexible we start to become in the way we practice and/or teach. If we teach or practice from a very rigid place, then our practice or teachings also become very rigid. A confused, rigid mind prevents us from going deeper. The more we sit down to do the meditation practices that Mikao Usui introduced in his teachings, the more open and flexible our mind will become, which in turn will have an effect on how we teach and practice.

It is said that Mikao Usui taught his students according to their spiritual progress. The openness that we find in consistent meditation practice lays bare our innate wisdom and compassion, qualities that we need in order to teach each person according to his/her spiritual progress. No open mind means no wisdom and compassion to teach or to practice in a fluid way.

That Mikao Usui would have taught in this way makes perfect sense as this really is how all the masters of old were teaching as well. Shakyamuni Buddha taught different teachings to different people depending on their state of mind. Everybody is in a uniquely different place along his or her path at any given time. So we cannot teach everybody in exactly the same way, for in doing this, we create rigid systems and rigid mindsets.

In the beginning we will copy the teacher so that we slowly start to understand the technique. But the more we practice the technique the more we will make it our own. It becomes more organic in relation to each person, as both teacher and student travel along their respective paths, meeting each other where they are at that time.

> When the mind resides in technique, chi is hindered and is not in harmony.
> – Issai Chozanshi, *The Demon's Sermon on the Martial Arts*

For example, say you teach a person hands-on healing. After a long time of practice, the student will start to flow more organically from her own open expanded state of mind, moving away from rigid hand-positions and away from any desire to judge or critique what is happening during a hands-on healing session. An open expanded state of mind/heart lets the student leave behind the idea that, for example, heat means this or that, an idea that depends solely on the perception of the person teaching it. The deeper we go the more we will find our own way into this, not in the rigid protocol of belief systems.

> Although you and I share the same biological architecture and function, perhaps what I perceive as a distinct color and smell is not exactly equal to the color and smell you perceive. We may give the same name to similar perceptions, but we cannot know how they relate to the reality of the outside world. Perhaps we never will.
> – Dr. Jorge Martins de Oliveira, Director of the Department of Neurosciences of the Institute of Human Being

In his precepts, Mikao Usui also pointed out flexibility and teaching people according to their spiritual progress.

Do not anger
Do not worry
Be grateful
Practice diligently
Show compassion to yourself and others

Let's take a look at the precept: practice diligently. The Japanese sentence is: Gyō o hageme, 業 を はけめ. This can be directly translated as practice diligently. However, the word gyō can mean so much more.

Hiroshi Doi translates this phrase as, "Do what you are meant to do." And yet another translation is: "Be true to your way and your being."

Dai Ajari Ryōjun Shionuma, who in Japan is seen as a living Buddha, points out that gyō can mean many different things:

> I would like at this point to reflect on what "practice" or "gyō" means in this context. For some, gyō means a special period of time of one-hundred or one-thousand days, but for others gyō is more of a lifetime activity or, more precisely, a way of life. Furthermore, for some, gyō is undertaken with the aim to reform oneself, and thus is seen as a self-centered activity. In contrast, others understand gyō as being performed for the benefit of other sentient beings, and is thus seen as an altruistic activity. In short, there are many different ways to understand what gyō really is.

For me, gyō is being true to my way and my being, not to someone else's way but to my own organic nature. But we really can only start to embody this when we let go of our anger and worry. Because if we anger and worry we cannot be flexible; we cannot be true to our way and our being.

According to the *Dictionary of Buddhism*, gyō 業 also can mean "activity" and "pure experience." This activity from a pure experience is an activity from our true self. An activity from pure experience is when we are free and can flow within the flow of the universe, instead of being stuck with man-made rigid rules.

Thus as we can see through these translations of gyō 業, Mikao Usui pointed out within the precepts the idea of practicing and teaching from a state of mind of flexibility. Ultimately we have to learn how to be true to our own pure organic experience and not to the teacher's experiences. The teacher is only there to help us find our own inner free-flowing organic pure experience, with our own inner light pointing out the way.

Chapter 53

Be True to Your Way and Your True Self

Often teachings can become too strict, with too many rules laid down by the teacher. When teachings become too strict, we can't move in the open expanded spacious flow of universal energy. Instead we are bound by rules and boxed in by ideas and concepts. At this stage, our practice becomes stiff instead of flowing. These rules, labels and concepts also mean that our practice cannot move into the organic way of our true self.

If we follow strict rules and concepts a teacher has laid down, we are following the teacher's experiences. But the teacher's experiences might be very different from ours. Maybe the teacher likes a specific way of placing the hands during a hands-on healing session. Suddenly these hand positions become a must and you start to question yourself: if you do not place your hands exactly as the teacher did, will your hands-on healing sessions "not work"?

Or, if the teacher feels heat and interprets that it means this or that, suddenly that becomes the standard interpretation. Or, the teacher might not like the color black and follows a rule that when you do hands-on healing you should wear only white or light colors. But all of these are the teacher's experiences and not yours. The teacher is there not to imprint his experiences on you, but to help you to find your own fluid experience.

However, if we just do what comes into our monkey mind, then we are just making things up. And maybe that is not helpful at all for ourselves or for our client. Thus there needs to be balance between firm and flexible, or in other words, between stable common sense and being in the flow.

Being in the flow means that the flow comes from our true self. This in turn means that to be in the flow takes time and practice, as it takes time and practice to really tap into our true self. Let me point it out again because this is very important: the flow does not come from our confused mind full of worry, fear, anger and attachment. This flow is the true flow from our true self.

Let's look at the precepts, in which we can see these teachings:

Do not anger
Do not worry
Be grateful
Be true to your way and your true self
Show compassion to yourself and others

The precept "be true to your way and your true self" is an important reminder. This precept in Japanese is "Gyō o hageme" which often has been translated as "work hard," "work honestly," or "practice diligently." However, there is a wonderful depth to the word gyō 業.

Gyō can mean work, patience, karma and pure experience.

This pure experience means knowledge derived from the direct experience of our true self.

Hiroshi Doi translates this precept as: "Do what you are meant to do." But to do that, this "doing" needs to come from our true self. Thus at a deeper level gyō o hageme means "be true to your way and your true self." If we look at the precepts, we can see that to be true to our way and our being we have to let go of our worry, fear, and anger, and be grateful for all that we encounter. Hence it is not that easy to step into the flow.

Thus the teacher is there to help you to be true to your way and your true self, not to box you in with her/his ways. The more we get boxed in with a teacher's way, the harder it is for us to remember our own way and to be true to our true self.

A good teacher therefore will adjust each student's practice according to the student's experience, state of mind, and physique. For example, the practice of a novice student with a racing, stress-filled mind and arthritic knees will be very different from an experienced student with a relaxed mind who is able to kneel or sit cross-legged for long periods of time. In making appropriate recommendations and adjustments to your practice, your teacher slowly helps to lay bare your true self, your Reiki. And in this way, now your practice starts to flow from your true self.

Chapter 54

Discovering Your Own Innate Healing Power

A real teacher isn't doing the healing for you. Instead she creates a space in which you can rediscover your own innate healing power.

Real healing is about rediscovering your own innate power. Often we give this power away to a practitioner or a teacher. We start to rely on them. They will make us better, or they will do some magical ritual and suddenly we are enlightened. But we all know that this is just an illusion; it doesn't work that way. Often we want it that way because it means we do not have to do anything at all; the practitioner or the teacher will do the hard work for us. However, it is a lazy way out and this kind of thinking leaves us un-empowered.

A real teacher helps us to find that innate power within us again. She will teach us how to empower ourselves, and how to discover what we have forgotten, our own innate healing power.

However, if the teacher doesn't know how to access his own innate healing power, then it will be very difficult for him to help us to rediscover ours.

But what is this innate healing power in the first place?

The real innate healing power is our true self in its fullest because in this state we are so open and expanded, like space. And thus we have a tremendous amount of free-flowing energy.

When we remember our true self, our mind has become clear like a mirror. Thus the teacher holds up the mirror of her true self and therefore we can see very clearly our own true self in the reflection. But if the mirror is dusty with attachments, ego, worry, anger, fear, then we cannot see anything at all. We might just get a small glimmer of our true self, of our own innate power to heal ourselves, but that is it. Thus it is of utmost importance that the practitioner or teacher makes sure the mirror of their own mind is crystal clear. Else there is nothing to show.

When the mirror is not clear, a teacher might even start to enforce in us the codependent idea that only he or she can do it for you. It might even feel as if they take your power away, instead of empowering you.

Thus the clearer the teacher's mind is, the clearer the space she can create – a clear space in which we can remember our own innate healing power.

Chapter 55

Reiju – Giving and Receiving, Together as One

Reiju (Japanese kanji 霊授) is one of the essential elements within the system of Reiki. Literally it means spiritual blessing or offering.

Often this is seen as a one-way experience from teacher to student, with the student being the one who is benefiting from, receiving something from this Reiju. However, I never have taught it this way because for me it is a union, a union of the teacher, student, and the universe. And from this union, experience, Reiju, all will benefit.

The kanji of ju (授) points this out as well. Ju is mostly translated as "to give."

But Zen Master Jakusho Kwong, in his book *No Beginning, No End: The Intimate Heart of Zen*, states that: "This word ju [授] is very good. 'To cut,' 'to open,' 'to empty,' and 'to receive' are all expressed by ju." For me these words describe exactly what I experience when I perform a Reiju. The empty state of mind, the experience that I also receive at the same time, and that the whole process is about openness because the ego temporarily is cut away. I wanted to investigate this a bit more.

I consulted a Japanese friend who is an international calligraphist and who looks deeply into kanji and its meanings. She came back with a wonderful explanation that put the phrase "receiving Reiju" in a whole new light.

The kanji 授 means "Receive" which is used when you receive

something very special and very valuable (but you can't buy) from god or respectable people (even nature). Just regular kanji for "receive" is 受.

Her explanation made so much sense because during Reiju both teacher and student receive "grace of the universe," "grace of our true self," "grace of nature," which is very special and very valuable indeed. This grace of course is unification, which the Oxford Dictionary defines as the "process of being united or made into a whole." So the word "receive" is not to be taken literally. It is an expedient means to a simple explanation of Reiju.

The deepest state of Reiju is that there is nothing to receive, nothing to give, and no gift. This is symbolized by the kanji of Rei 霊 – spiritual.

To sum this all up: when performing a spiritual (Rei 霊) blessing (Ju 授), the teacher is giving and receiving at the same time. Therefore this also means that for a teacher performing Reiju is a spiritual meditative practice for remembering one's own true self.

Now we can start to see why Shinpiden Reiki Level III is not just about becoming a teacher. It is about learning to empower yourself through performing Reiju. Shinpiden (meaning "mystery teachings") is all about rediscovering the mystery of our non-dual state of mind where receiving and giving happens simultaneously, where "teacher" and "student" are receiving and giving, together as one.

Part 7

The Path to Healing

Chapter 56

The Stepping Stones

Within the system of Reiki there are many stepping stones, however, the first few are all about ourselves. Shoden Reiki I is foremost about meditating on the precepts, practicing the meditation practices like jōshin kokyū hō and seishin toitsu and hands-on healing on yourself. It is out of this that comes hands-on healing on others. Hands-on healing on others is in fact one of the last stepping stones as it needs to come from the space of our own clear mind: a mind of no anger or worry, of being humble, honest and compassionate. This way hands-on healing becomes like a moving meditation; we are mindful during the session, which means we can slip into our non-dual state of mind much more easily.

The next stepping stone is Okuden Reiki II in which we start to deepen this mindfulness through meditating on the symbols, chanting the mantras and with the meditation practice of hatsurei hō. Again this is all for ourselves. Okuden means inner or hidden teachings so the tools taught within this level are all about rediscovering what is hidden inside of us: our true self/Reiki. When we start to rediscover our true self, our innate great bright light starts to become brighter and brighter, and we can use this light for performing hands-on healing on others. The more we start to rediscover our true self, the more we start to go into this non-dual, mindfulness state and the deeper hands-on healing for others will be. We can now start to see the reasons why Mikao Usui added these stepping stones within his system, slowly moving forward to rediscovering our true self.

Within Shinpiden Reiki III, we start to go even deeper into rediscovering our true self. Shinpiden means mystery teachings, which are pointing us to the mystery of our true self, the mystery of Reiki. In these teachings we start to realize that the hands are only a very small part of the system of Reiki, that in fact our whole body emanates light. At this stage we start to rediscover that we can be Reiki – be our true self – be the great bright light, in all we do. This in turn means that we can bring healing into our daily life more and more. We cannot walk in the street and say to each person we come across, "Excuse me, can I do hands-on healing on you." They would probably think we are mad! But we can walk in this state of mind of great bright light, emanating a field of compassion and wisdom from which each person, animal, tree, etc who comes in contact with this field can take whatever he or she needs for healing to take place. This field is a field of embodiment of the precepts, a field of no anger, no worry, being humble and grateful, honest, and compassionate. This emanation of the great bright light of our true self is a way of touching others so much more deeply than just with the hands. It is a way of Being, a way of Life. This state of being Reiki, our true self, is the last stepping stone. However, this last stepping stone is bringing us back to the first stepping stone and we travel the path again, and again, like an Enso, the Zen circle: no beginning, no end.

Chapter 57

Healing is Preparation

Healing is not just about going to a practitioner when you don't feel well. Healing is not just about using self-healing practices at the moment you get sick. Healing is about starting right here, right in this current moment. Healing is about nurturing balance and harmony not just in our bodies, but also in our minds and hearts. Healing is all about preparing ourselves for when we do get sick, or when our marriage falls apart, or when there is a natural disaster. If we wait to start our spiritual practice until we are unwell or when things are difficult, we might not have the energy and commitment to perform a meditation practice, or we might feel too tired or overwhelmed by our issues. But right here, right in this moment, when you feel all is going okay in your life, you have the energy to practice. *The Yellow Emperor's Classic of Medicine* (considered the ancient authority on Chinese medicine) stated this wonderfully:

> Listen, treating a disease that has already developed, or trying to bring order to disruptions that have already begun, is like digging a well after you've become thirsty, or making weapons after the battle is over. Wouldn't it already be too late?

This means that real healing is a preparation practice; it helps us to build a strong foundation within ourselves so that we do not get overwhelmed or carried away by all our emotions when we face difficulties in our lives. The best way to prepare is to begin today with practices that strengthen the spirit, balance the heart, and calm the mind.

Chapter 58

Ultimate Healing Starts in Our Mind/heart

It is only through remembering our true self that healing will last forever.

Many people talk about healing but what is it really?

Healing is about becoming whole, remembering what we have forgotten. Becoming whole doesn't always mean the removal of the symptoms; rather it is about how to live with the symptoms in a wholesome way.

What we have forgotten is our true self, our essence. Remembering our essence is therefore the real healing. When we remember our true self we start to feel less angry, less worried and fearful, and we become more compassionate to ourselves and others. Therefore, real healing not only will have an effect on yourself but also on your family, your community, and the world as a whole.

Real healing therefore takes place in our mind/heart! This is why all the old spiritual traditions mention specific states of mind/heart which need to be healed, like ignorance, anger, attachments, hatred, greed, etc.

However, in many modern healing methods we seem to have forgotten this and we focus most of the time just on the physical aspect of healing. In doing this, we forget that the real healing takes place in our mind/heart.

Don't get me wrong; physical healing is wonderful. But we also know that we cannot take our physical body with us when the time comes for us to leave the physical world. Plus when we get older we often have more aches and pains, and most of us become more fragile. This means that we cannot always cure physical issues, due to the natural process of our body's aging. However, we still can have a wholesome state of mind/heart. And if we have a wholesome state of mind/heart, we will look at our physical issues from a very different perspective.

The more we start to remember our true self, the more we step into the realm of real healing. At this stage we will not get caught up in the melodrama of our physical issues; we can start to accept them more openly. And by accepting these physical issues more openly, we have more energy for physical healing to happen! The more we complain about our issues, the more we are angry and worried about them, the more constrained we become, the less energy flows freely through us to help us heal physical issues. Therefore it is paramount that if we want to heal ourselves physically, we first need to heal our mind/heart.

Our true self is always whole, always bright, perfect, and in union with the universe. If we remember this, then all our physical issues do not have any power over us; this way we do not define ourselves by our physical self or get distracted by our physical self. Our body dies, but our true self lasts forever and thus when we remember our true self, we let go of our biggest fear: fear of death. And this in turn again softens our physical issues. This again is the real healing for which we need to strive.

Nowadays there are many modalities which focus on "healing" others on a physical level, yet they forget to help the client to empower themselves to start to remember their true self. It is in remembering the true self that real healing can take place. But of course the practitioner or teacher only can do this if they are willing to look first at healing their own mind/heart. We cannot help others to rediscover their true self if we as practitioners and teachers still are fumbling around in the dark.

Therefore real healing takes place directly within ourselves; direct healing within ourselves will indirectly help others.

Chapter 59

We Can Only Heal Ourselves

Healing ourselves is something we can only do ourselves. While we can be told this again and again, we need to rediscover it for ourselves. And because most of the time we look for healing outside of ourselves, most of the time we find it hard to accept that all we need for healing actually is inside of us already. Healing means to make whole; this in essence is about rediscovering our true self, our inner bright light. Therefore, healing is not about curing. Curing happens when we go to a doctor and the doctor performs an operation to fix a knee problem, for example. Healing goes much deeper, to the essence of our being; it is about our mind/heart.

All the teachings of old point out that we need to look within and that real healing is not to be found externally.

> The kingdom of God is within you.
> – Luke 17:21

Of course sometimes we need external help to guide us in the right direction because we are so lost and do not know where to look or how to look within. But the external help is not there to save us or to do all the work for us. This external help is just there to guide us in the direction of looking within so that we can start to heal ourselves, heal ourselves from the inside out.

When someone comes for a healing session with me, the first thing I point out is that they need to set their intention to heal themselves. I remind them that I am just a facilitator to help them rediscover their own innate healing power, which they have had – which we all have – since conception. But often we forget this because within our society we look so externally. When we start to remember this innate healing power, we feel an inner strength, an inner power source, which we can utilize during our busy, chaotic daily life.

This kind of healing doesn't always mean we will be cured. But even if issues we may have are not cured, we will start to deal with our issues in a much better way because we have a calmer more open state of mind/heart.

This kind of healing is also about self-responsibility. Within the system of Reiki we often hear that all we need is a reiju/initiation/ attunement and presto! We can channel the universe in all its clarity. But if we think and look honestly, we know this is not really the case. The first issue with this idea is that we say we need to "channel" the energy; we see it somewhere outside of us. But take a clear look and notice that we are not outside of the universe. Rather, we are smack bang in the middle of it; in fact we ARE it. The essence of the universe is as much within as it is without/ outside, which means we do not have to channel it at all. We just have to realize that we are it: We Are The Universe. But this kind of realization is not easy to come by, and this is why Mikao Usui put meditation practices within his teachings.

By practicing these meditations, we realize we have a responsibility to remember our union with the universe, with God, with Buddha. This in fact is our innate healing power. And by remembering this innate healing power, we can start to genuinely heal ourselves.

Chapter 60

Let Go of Labelling, Distinguishing, and Judging

The more we try to interpret an experience and clothe it in words, the more we remove ourselves from it. We are left with "fixed" concepts, and a dualistic view concerning the world, so our responses and reactions to daily situations do not flow from a natural state.
– Tarthang Tulku, *Openness Mind*

Why is it so important in our modern world to let go of labelling, distinguishing, and judging?

One of the reasons why we have so many conflicts in our world is that we constantly label, distinguish, and judge. There is no harmony, no balance, no flow from our natural state, our true self.

Labelling, distinguishing, and judging is done because we constantly are comparing. Comparing what is good or bad, comparing what is smelly or not, comparing what is hot or cold, comparing, comparing, and comparing. Our constant monkey mind of comparing never seems to stop. This in itself will deplete our energy over time, creating a tired, stressful, closed-minded state of mind.

When we compare we create trouble, and this kind of trouble might end up in not being compassionate to others and even to ourselves.

But when you do not observe the thought carefully, you may find yourself labelling or judging the experience. When this happens you will not be contacting the deeper, more subtler levels of the experience, and your awareness will be somewhat superficial.

– Tarthang Tulku, *Openness Mind*

Let's take a closer look. We might say, "The tree I see in my garden is tall." But is it? How do I know it is tall? Because I compare it with something else.

Yes, compared to the small bush next to it the tree is indeed tall. But compared to the big mountain behind it the tree is small. So what is the tree, tall or small? Neither! It is just a tree and that is all.

The more we compare, the more we label, distinguish, and judge. But what would happen if we stop all of that? If we see things simply for what they are, what would take place? We would see the tree just as a tree, neither tall, ugly, beautiful, just a tree. We would see a person just for what they are, neither ugly nor beautiful; we would see the experience for what it is, neither good nor bad. This in turn creates a sense of gratefulness for each experience we encounter.

This kind of seeing without labelling, distinguishing, and judging creates compassion. Most of the time we have limited compassion because instead we choose to use comparisons. We compare, label, distinguish, and judge someone as nice or not nice, someone as ugly or pretty, someone as stinky or pleasant smelling. Thus, even if we want to help someone, we gravitate towards the things we like and not towards the things we dislike.

Thus labelling, distinguishing, and judging creates duality: things we like and do not like. This in turn will create attachments to things we like and we will push away things we do not like. And to take that a step further we now have sown the seeds of anger, worry, jealousy... We get worried when the person who we do not like asks for our help; we get angry when the stinky person is asking something from us; we become jealous when someone else is talking to our beautiful friend.

As we now start to see, labelling, distinguishing, and judging is a breeding ground for anger, worry, fear and jealousy, just to name a few. Do these traits sound familiar?

This is why any serious spiritual practice is all about letting go of labelling, distinguishing, and judging, because that way we can become compassionate human beings. This in turn will create a compassionate world in which we see equanimity and harmony. Choose compassion over comparison. Choose compassion over categorizing.

> For whenever we are involved in categorizing or interpreting, the mind cuts itself off from the experience, causing us to become caught up in an endless progression of thoughts.
> – Tarthang Tulku, *Openness Mind*

Chapter 61

The Wow Moment in Reiki

When you walk around a corner and you suddenly see an amazing architectural work like, for example, the Sagrada Familia church in Barcelona, all you can say is, "Wow!" You are speechless, no need for words: just, "Wow!"

After the initial Wow moment you start to explain it in words to the person next to you, but these words cannot even describe your initial response. Your initial "Wow!" was a whole body/mind/ energy experience, beyond words. As you explain your Wow experience in words to your friend, you might start to look at individual elements of the church, and this takes you even further away from the whole initial experience of the Wow moment. By looking at each individual element, we start to miss the whole.

This is the same as when we try to describe a hands-on healing session or a reiju/initiation/attunement; the initial Wow moment is the most important. That is the Reiki experience that is beyond words, beyond focusing on each specific element of the session; it is all encompassing.

When we perform a hands-on healing session we need to try to stay in this Wow moment in each moment of the whole session. As soon as we think, "Now I feel this" or "Now my client needs that," then we have already moved away from the openness of the Wow moment. When we are in the Wow moment there is no "I," there is no "you," there is just "Wow!" As soon as we focus on a specific area and we say for example, "I need to draw this symbol," then the "I" has come into play. We can see this also when we try to explain what we felt during a treatment. We might say, "I felt this or that" or "I saw this or that" or "I think you need this or that." These statements are all about the "I" or the ego. If we only could stay in the initial Wow moment then we would realize that, in reality, there is no "I." We do not say, "I Wow"; we just say, "Wow!"

The Wow moment happens before we start to label things, like when we walk around that corner and see that amazing church Sagrada Familia in Barcelona; all we can do is say, "Wow!" because we haven't labelled the church as of yet. In this Wow moment we are unified with the church and unified with the universe, because we haven't separated the church, the universe and the "I" yet. Wow. Just Wow.

When we have the Wow moment during a hands-on healing session or a reiju/initiation/attunement, we are one with our client or student. There is nothing to interpret, nothing to explain, nothing to do; just "Wow!" This of course is also the case for the client or student, who also have their Wow moment. But as soon as they start to describe what they felt or experienced, the initial Wow moment is gone, and we are separated again.

The aim within the system of Reiki is to be in this wonder of the Wow moment not just during Reiki treatments or practice, but in every moment of every day. When we awaken to the reality that every moment of our lives contains the whole universe, we will find ourselves saying, "Wow!"

Chapter 62

Jumping into the Stream of Our Confused Thinking

Our true self is always clear, bright, compassionate and full of wisdom. But often we seem to focus more on our confused mind than on our true self, due to the habits we have formed over time.

We may have picked up these habits as kids through our parents, education, society, etc. Some habits are easy to let go of, as we hold them in an open hand. Others can be very hard to let go of, as we hold them in a clenched fist.

But we always have a choice whether to follow our habitual patterns or not.

Imagine these patterns like a stream: the mind stream of worry, fear, anger, jealousy, just to name a few. We can choose to jump into the stream of worry and if this stream is habitually very strong, it can carry us away very quickly. It feels like we are being carried away further and further from our true self. And if we stay in this stream of our confused mind, eventually it may become a river with a stronger current to carry us away further still. But if we investigate this through meditation practices, we come to the conclusion that all we have to do is climb out of the confused mind streams and we will find that our true self is there. Of course, to do this is not so easy. But no matter where and when we climb out of the stream, our true self is there.

The more we practice meditations, the more clearly we can start to recognize these kinds of individual confused mind streams into which we jump daily. And the more clearly we start to see these confused mind streams, the more clearly we can see our choices. We can choose to jump into them and get carried away in the current, or we can choose to stay in the space of our true self, full of compassion and wisdom. Thus the more we remember our true self, the more aware we become of the different streams of thinking. When we stay with these moments of awareness, these moments of our true self, we feel less need to jump into the stream of our confused thinking.

Often we may feel that we need to stay in the stream of our confused thinking because that is how we "I"dentify ourselves. And when we climb out of this stream we feel we start to lose our "I"dentity. We are the worrier, the angry one, or the jealous one; we have been conditioned that way. Therefore it can be scary to climb out of the river of our conditioned thinking and onto the bank of our true self because we have to change the way we are used to thinking about ourselves. Our confused mind may tell us again and again that change is scary. But as soon as we are on the bank of our true self, we feel we can finally let go of our mistaken "I"dentity. We finally feel free. This means that when something triggers our worry, fear, or jealousy, we do not have to follow our habitual jumping in to that specific mind stream, and therefore we do not get carried away anymore. We can stay stable, free, and open on the bank of our true self.

Imagine again our mind patterns like a stream and remember how we may see our habits – easy to let go of as we hold them in an open hand or hard to let go of as we hold them in a clenched fist. If we are in a stream, flailing away with clenched fists, do we get anywhere? Not likely. We may splash and stir up the water a bit, but we will stay stuck in the same small space. But if instead we open our hands, minds, and hearts, moving into the flow of the stream, we either can paddle forward or float back to the bank of our true self much more easily. Again, practicing meditations helps us to recognize our mind patterns and habits, and helps us to see our choices.

But if we do fall into the stream, instead of flailing around and getting stuck in anger, worry, or "I"dentity, let's instead choose to go with the flow of gratitude and compassion, climb back out onto the bank and into the light of our true self.

Chapter 63

The Mirror of Our Mind

Our True Identity is like a crystal-clear mirror.

However, most of the time our mirror-like mind is covered with dust – the dust of attachments, worry, anger, and jealousy, just to name a few. To clean the mirror we turn to our daily meditation practices, which sounds easy. But this is not always the case.

Imagine we have a cloth and we wipe the mirror clean. Now look at the cloth; it is all dirty from the layers of dust that were accumulated on the mirror. Therefore in our meditation practices, we might first get a bit dirty as all the old dust, which has been sitting there for ages, gets stirred up. In the beginning we might label this dirt as bad. But in fact, if we label it as bad, we start to get caught up with the dust, and therefore, the dust falls back on the mirror again.

Even if there are many layers of dust on our mirror-like mind, look beyond the dust; look at the mirror itself. The mirror-like mind can reflect everything, yet it never labels or judges. It just reflects everything as it is. Thus when the dust is stirred up and we get covered in some of the dust, let's let go of labelling it bad or good. Just accept it as it is, like the mirror. If we simply accept the dust as it is, it will melt like snow in the blazing sun, and suddenly we can gain an insight into our True Identity.

By rediscovering our mirror-like mind, we start to live a life free from labelling and judging, which means our life will be full of inner joy and happiness. Because it is through labelling and judging that we get caught up in the dust.

But even if we wipe away the dust of our mirror-like mind in one big sweep, new daily dust keeps falling on our mirror. Therefore, we still have to keep on with our regular meditation practices, our daily dusting, so to speak.

What else happens when we have rediscovered the crystal-clear mirror of our mind?

Other people can start to see the reflection of their True Identity in it. Of course the other person needs to have a reasonably clear mirror as well, or else nothing will be reflected at all. But even one little gap within the dust can reflect the clarity of our True Identity. Place one crystal-clear mirror opposite a dusty mirror that has one little clear patch in it. Within that one little clear patch, we can start to see the reflection of everything else within the other, clear mirror. Thus by remembering our own crystal-clear mirror-like mind, we start to sow the seed for a world of wisdom and compassion, a world where wisdom and compassion can be reflected to infinity.

Chapter 64

Letting Go of the "I"

The whole system of Reiki is about letting go of the "I." Mikao Usui pointed this out very clearly within the precepts.

Do not be angry
Do not worry
Be grateful
Practice this diligently
Show compassion to yourself and others

If we look to the precepts only at a superficial level, we will not see that they are about letting go of the "I." But if we look within them more deeply, we can see this clearly. Let's ask ourselves some questions and see what the answers are.

Who gets angry?
I get angry.
Who gets worried?
I get worried.
Who is not being grateful?
I am not being grateful.

Who is in the way of not practicing diligently?
I am in the way of not practicing diligently.

Who is in the way of being compassionate?
I am in the way of being compassionate.

Looking at it from a deeper perspective, slowly we can start to see that the precepts therefore are about letting go of the "I." If we let go of the "I" then there is no "I" who gets angry or worried. There is no "I" who is in the way of being grateful, not practicing diligently, or being compassionate.

However, it seems that within many teachings of the system of Reiki, often we try to strengthen the grip on the "I," rather than gradually (and maybe one day completely) letting go of the "I."

Let's look at an example of doing hands-on healing on others.

When we feel something while doing hands-on healing on others, often we start to label what we feel; we might feel something and label it heat, for example. As soon as we label it heat we might say to ourselves, "Because I feel the heat, now I need to use this symbol." Or we might say: "Because I feel heat this means that my client has a serious issue."

Labelling, distinguishing, and judging all come from the "I" – I feel this and therefore I will do that to my client. Aside from the fact that we are "doing" rather than "being," by labelling, distinguishing, and judging, we tighten our grip on the "I." So we also can ask ourselves some simple questions: Who is labelling? Who is distinguishing? Who is judging? The answer to all of these is "I am."

Mikao Usui also added mindfulness practices within his teaching, like jōshin kokyū hō, or focusing on a mantra or symbol.

> Mindfulness requires observation, but it must be free from interpretation and passing judgement.
> – Tarthang Tulku, *Openness Mind*

These mindfulness practices are there also to help us let go of the "I" so that we can reach the ultimate teachings within the system of Reiki: just Be.

When we just Be with our client we start to go into a state of oneness which cannot happen when the "I" is involved. Because as soon as there is an "I," there is a "me" and a "you" and suddenly we are separate.

To be Reiki is the essence of Mikao Usui's teachings, but to just Be we have to let go of the "I."

Does letting go of the "I" mean that we lose our unique humanness – say, our beliefs, our beautiful singing voice, our love of chocolate ice cream? – and become a bland, nameless, faceless person with no opinions as we go through our life?

No; it simply means that we let go of attachments to thoughts like, "I am a kinder person than you because I have been practicing for 5 years and you only just started," "My voice is more pleasant to listen to than yours because I have perfect pitch," or "I have a more sophisticated palate than you because I like chocolate and you like vanilla." While each of these – comparing, labelling, distinguishing, judging – may be true to our human mind, they all create separateness.

And separateness – holding on to "I" and "you" – is like trying to hold on to a cloud, something temporary that will come and go. If, instead, we practice mindfulness "free from interpretation and passing judgment," if we practice the system of Reiki in that way, we can begin to loosen our grip on the "I" and hold on to something that always was and is with us: our true self. In doing this, we can just Be.

Part 8

The Nature of Reiki

Chapter 65

Reiki and Nature

For me the system of Reiki is about rediscovering our true self, which we also could call our True Nature. Our True Nature indicates that we need to realign ourselves with the natural elements.

Nature is always in harmony; nature doesn't judge, label or distinguish. Nature flows, and is therefore about becoming natural. We have lost our natural ways, hiding them underneath all our pretending, our masks, our attachments, our fears and worries. Thus, to become natural again we need to let go of these layers and let our true nature, our true self, our Reiki, shine.

Mikao Usui pointed out how important the natural elements are within his teachings. However, we have to look deeply into the teachings to see this.

Here are just a few examples of what we can find in Mikao Usui's teachings, and the interconnectedness with nature.

Deep within the word Reiki we see rain; this represents the idea that we just need to let go and absorb the spiritual rain which is always falling. Rain doesn't label, judge, or distinguish; it just rains, and the earth takes from it what it needs. When we practice, either for ourselves or with others, what if we just let it rain? No need to say, "You need this or that energy," "You need this or that symbol," "You need this and not that, let me take it out." Just let it rain.

Within the Reiki III symbol/mantra dai kômyô, we can see the sun and the moon. The sun and moon also do not judge, label, or distinguish; they just shine and everything takes from them accordingly. Sun and moon are also about balance and harmony and compassion and wisdom.

Within the kanji of Ki, we see mist or vapor. For most of us, our energy is more like frozen water, stuck everywhere due to all our worries, fears, anger, and attachments. But when we start to practice and become more open, our energy becomes like mist: fluid, soft and yet able to penetrate everywhere. This is why when we as practitioners have laid bare this mist-like energy, we only have to touch one part of the body for the energy to penetrate the body like mist.

Within Reiju we again can see the rain, and this time we see the rain which falls internally: our inner blessings. This rain is what they often call amrita in esoteric traditions. The deeper we go within our practice, the more we start to feel this internal rain falling down and blessing our whole being.

If we look deeply within the Okuden Reiki II mantras, we can see fire and water.

This fire melts our frozen energy so that it can be flowing like water. And if we heat up/deepen our practice enough, this water becomes mist or vapor which in turn becomes rain. It is the natural cycles which we need to realize internally. The universe is us and we are the universe. And to rediscover this, we need to see that deep within us we have the same cycles as the universe. This is really what Mikao Usui was pointing out in his teachings.

These are just a few examples of the hidden inner teachings of Mikao Usui's system. But as teachers, we can only really teach this if we have had direct experiences of these natural elements within ourselves. Otherwise, it just becomes an intellectual teaching with no foundation of the direct experience. Meditating on the precepts, meditating with hands-on healing, meditating on the symbols and mantras, the meditation practices like jōshin kokyū hō and the moving meditation of Reiju – all of these are practices which can bring the direct experience of the natural elements into our own being.

Chapter 66

In Harmony with Nature

... yamabushi training takes place in the middle of nature. Simply, it is to connect ourselves back to nature.
– Fumihiro Hoshino, Shugendo Priest

It is said that Mikao Usui was a Shugenja/yamabushi, a practitioner who walks in the mountains to realize harmony with the natural elements. When we walk in nature with an open mind/heart we can start to feel how we need to practice the system of Reiki; more than that, we begin to realize how we need to lead our lives. Nature shows us how to live in harmony, but in modern times we have removed ourselves so far from nature that sometimes it is hard to see what nature is teaching us.

As practitioners of the system of Reiki, we try to make our internal energy flow again as it has become stagnant over time due to things like fear, worry, anger and more. When our energy flows, our mind/heart also starts to flow and is more at ease with what is happening in life. If we think about – or better yet, watch – water, we can see that Nature is showing this to us: if water in a river is partly frozen and it hits a rock, it will hit the rock again and again over and over. If the water is completely melted it flows freely around any rock or obstacle. Nature is showing us how to be more free flowing; it is telling us to practice until our energy and mind/heart are like free running water.

As human beings, we are animals on the move in search of food, and this is what makes the fountain of life possible. However, plants search for food simply by placing themselves in nature. Plants can get vital energy from the space around them as well

as above and below them just by being situated in nature. That is what it means by being there. I think yamabushi practices are really close to this – placing oneself in nature.
– Fumihiro Hoshino, Shugendo Priest

By placing ourselves in nature, we can illuminate the best way to approach our Reiki practice. Many Reiki teachings are very strict with hand positions or how to do a specific practice, teaching that it cannot be done any other way. Does this strictness follow the way of nature? If we look at nature, we can see that nature is both firm and flexible at the same time.

Let's look at the trees for example: the wind blows but each tree moves in its own unique way. No two trees move in exactly the same way. In an old tree, the trunk stands stable as the upper leaves and branches may sway in the wind; a very young tree in a strong wind may move almost top to bottom. But both trees are anchored by their roots. In the same way, we can see the wind as the energy that moves through and around us, and see the trees as us, the practitioners. So the best practice is to move in your own unique way, yet rooted in the foundation of the practice and teachings. To be more in harmony with nature, we need to let go of the strict rules some people apply when teaching. Yes, these rules are great as a foundation for our roots, but when we get higher into the teachings we become more and more flexible, like the tops of the trees gently swaying in their own unique way in harmony with the wind.

At the deepest level of Mikao Usui's teachings we will remember to "Be Reiki" instead of "Do Reiki." Again we can see this in nature, plants, trees and rocks: they are not thinking of Doing this or that. They are just Being. One rock doesn't say to the other rock, "I am jealous of you!" The rock is just Being. One tree doesn't say to the other tree, "You are taller than me and I do not like it!" The tree is just Being. The rain that falls on the forest is not saying, "You small plants, you need to receive this much rain (energy) and you big trees, you will receive this much rain (energy)!" The rain is just Being. A river is not saying to an obstacle that it comes across, "Get out of my way." The river is just Being.

So be in nature and let nature teach you the way back to your own True Nature.

Chapter 67

Our Inner Light

Often we look for healing outside of ourselves, for someone who can "fix" us or "heal" us. But in looking outside of ourselves, we give our own inner healing power away, leaving us unempowered instead of empowered. In essence, we can only heal ourselves; no one can do that for us, not even a Buddha. Someone can show us the way or can be a facilitator, but we still have to do the hard work ourselves.

I always see it like this: imagine that on the shadow side of a mountain, there is a dark cave. This represents our confused mind, a mind full of worry, anger, frustration, attachments, jealousy, you name it. The cave of our mind is dark because we haven't yet recognized our own inner luminosity.

Now imagine the sun, which represents the external factor for healing us; this might be a practitioner, a deity, or whatever we connect with when we think of the healing we seek. To find that healing, to dispel our darkness, we have to bring the sun into our cave each time. But after we have brought in the sun, the sun will go back again where it came from, leaving our mind dark once more. We feel good for a short moment when the sun is lighting up our dark mind, but as soon as the sun goes back home the light diminishes.

But what if we start to delve deeper into our own essence and start to rediscover our inner luminosity, our inner sun? Now we do not have to rely on an external factor anymore and our confused, dark cave-mind is lit up 24 hours a day. By rediscovering our own inner luminosity we start to empower ourselves; we are healing our own wounds. This gives us inner strength through which we can maintain our equilibrium during difficult times.

On the deepest level we need to realize that the cave and the sun are the same, that we are Buddha and Buddha is us. This is the state of mind of non-duality and in this state of mind our inner luminosity is always bright, always shining. No need to rely on any outer source anymore, because inside we always can find, and be, our own light.

If we keep telling ourselves that only an external force can heal us, then we become dependent on that external force. And if we continue on in this way of thinking, in this cave-mind of darkness, it will be hard to become independent and stand on our own two feet, to stand in our own luminosity and not in someone else's. When we empower ourselves, we can help others to empower themselves as well. When we rediscover our own inner luminosity, we can guide others to find theirs.

Chapter 68

Spacious Mind Spacious Heart

In many spiritual traditions, the essence of the mind/heart is symbolized by space. But why is this?

Our true mind/heart is a union with the universe. The universe has no beginning or end and therefore our mind/heart is as spacious as the universe. Space is a great metaphor because nothing sticks to space, we cannot hurt space, space cannot be damaged, and it can accommodate everything and anything.

When, through daily meditation practice, we start to remember our own spacious mind/heart, we will therefore become more accommodating to everybody. This in turn will increase our compassion. Often we are only compassionate to our family and friends; we are in a way narrow-minded in our mind/heart. And as such, we cannot accommodate more people, let alone accommodate animals, trees, you name it.

But through consistent practice, our mind/heart will be so spacious that our compassion includes everything. Everything will become sacred and therefore everything will be treated with respect, kindness, compassion, and love.

Often people feel overwhelmed when helping or being compassionate to others, but that is because we do not have the energy which comes freely when our mind/heart is spacious. Imagine your mind/heart as spacious as the universe: everything is free flowing, and your energy is not stuck anymore by small-minded concepts, attachments, fears, worry and jealousy. We have a tremendous amount of free-flowing energy which we can utilize to be compassionate to everyone and everything, without feeling overwhelmed or burned out by our compassion.

And even if the person who we are compassionate to doesn't say "thank you," we will be okay with this. Most of the time we want something in return for being compassionate to others; however, that is not real compassion. When we want something back from the other, our giving has strings attached to it; the strings of the ego tie us to a narrow mind/heart. Real compassion has no strings attached at all – in fact we give with the mindset of a spacious mind/ heart: no giver, nothing to give, and no receiver. Because when we are as spacious as the universe, we have the direct experience that everything is part of this universe, oneness; hence, no giver, no gift, or receiver.

A spacious mind/heart is so important in our modern-day world, as we get upset by so many small things which come our way. This happens because we have a narrow mind/heart full of anger, worry, or fear, to name but a few emotions we can let ourselves get stuck in. But with a spacious mind/heart nothing sticks! It is all okay.

These are just a few examples of why old spiritual traditions used the metaphor for space when pointing out our true mind/ heart. However, if it is only an intellectual concept, then we do not embody this spaciousness. Therefore we need to meditate so that we can have a direct experience of our true spacious mind/heart. In doing this, we can bring this state of mind/heart into all we do in our daily life.

One of the Meiji Emperor's waka used by Usui Mikao, as translated by Hyakuten Inamoto, says:

Asamidori sumiwataritaru ohzorano
hiroki onoga kokoro to mogana.

As a great sky in clear light green
I wish my heart would be as vast.

As we contemplate these words, we can imagine our mind/ heart expanding to be as vast as the sky. And through consistent meditation practice, through direct experience, our spacious mind/heart will become as vast as the universe, extending true compassion, respect, kindness, and love to one and all, as all are One.

Chapter 69

Reiki is Love

When you love someone, the best thing you can offer is your presence. How can you love someone if you are not there?
– Thich Nhat Hanh, *Fear: Essential Wisdom for Getting Through the Storm*

It is all very simple: Reiki is Love.

But this kind of love is no ordinary love. No, it is love in its purest form. Love without any strings attached, love that gives with an open heart and mind. This love does not label, judge, or distinguish; this love is free of all of that. This kind of love sets you free. As Thich Nhat Hanh states, "How can you love someone if you are not there?" He is pointing out that love is mindfulness, because if we are distracted by the past, present, and future, these distractions mean that we are not there for the other person. In fact, if we are distracted by the past, present, and future, we are not even there for ourselves.

Mrs. Takata had many different names for Reiki: God power, universal force from the great divine spirit, true energy, the great life force radiating from the sun. All of these point towards love, pure love.

The word Reiki also is seen as our true self, because it is only by remembering our true self that we start to express our pure love without any strings attached to it. We therefore could say that pure love emanates from our true self like life force radiating from the sun.

You must love in such a way that the person you love feels free.
– Thich Nhat Hanh, *True Love: A Practice for Awakening the Heart*

In a way, it is so simple that Reiki is love, and yet it is so hard to understand in its fullest. It is so difficult to love someone in such a way that the person feels free, because often we bind the person with strings of attachments. This is why Mikao Usui taught specific meditation practices, like meditating on the precepts, meditating on the symbols and mantras, hands-on healing as meditation, breathing meditations, and the moving meditation of Reiju. These practices help us to loosen the strings of our attachments and to rediscover our pure love, our essence, our true self, so that we can love everybody and everything in a free-flowing way.

Often it is only when people suddenly feel they are losing their partner that they realize how much they love them. Then they cling on even tighter. But the more they grasp, the more the other person escapes them, and the more fragile the relationship becomes. So often we want happiness, but the very way we pursue it is so clumsy and unskillful that it brings only more sorrow. Usually we assume we must grasp in order to have that something that will ensure our happiness. We ask ourselves: "How can we possibly enjoy anything if we cannot own it?" How often attachment is mistaken for love! Even when the relationship is a good one, love can be spoiled by attachment with its insecurity, possessiveness, and pride; and then when love is gone, all you have left to show for it are the "souvenirs" of love, the scars of attachment.
– Sogyal Rinpoche, *The Tibetan Book of Living and Dying*

Love, pure love, is love with non-attachment, love with kindness, humility, mindfulness, and openness. It is all very simple: Reiki is Love.

Chapter 70

Reiki is Compassion

It is very simple yet so profound, and at the same time difficult to embody: Reiki is Compassion.

Often we try so much to define what Reiki is or what the system of Reiki is, but in reality we can just say one word: compassion.

Traditionally the word Reiki stands for "your true self," which is your innate great bright light. This light emanates a warmth, the warmth of compassion. This compassionate warmth is comforting, supportive, and healing in nature.

When we practice hands-on healing with others, it is not really that we do it with our hands. They are just the conduits; the real healing comes from compassion.

When we practice a reiju/initiation/attunement with someone, the blessing doesn't really come from the ritual; it comes from compassion.

When we start to heal ourselves, it is not really from all the different methods taught within the system of Reiki; they are just fingers pointing towards the moon. The real healing comes from compassion.

Why does healing come from compassion?

Compassion is healing because real compassion comes from an open heart and mind. This openness is like space; it encompasses everything, and nothing is excluded. Thus it is as spacious as the universe. This spaciousness, this universal compassion, is full of unlimited energetic potential.

Compassion also is healing in nature because in the state of mind of compassion we do not judge, label, or distinguish.

In this state of mind of compassion there is no giver, no gift, and no receiver. No need to do anything, no need to draw symbols, no need to invoke deities, no need to direct the energy, no need to give something: just to Be. What a freedom, what a spaciousness, how compassionate this is.

We therefore can say that hands-on healing on others comes from a compassionate mind/heart.

We therefore can say that reiju/initiation/attunement comes from a compassionate mind/heart.

We therefore can say that healing ourselves comes from a compassionate mind/heart.

So again, Reiki is compassion: simple, yet so difficult to embody.

This also is why it is the last precept, as each one builds on the foundation of the others.

Do not be angry
Do not worry
Be grateful
Practice this diligently
Show compassion to yourself and others

Mikao Usui pointed out within the precepts that before we can have real compassion for ourselves and others we need to let go of all our anger, all our worry, and be grateful for everything – "good" and "bad." By practicing this diligently, we will one day lay bare our true self, our innate pure compassionate heart and mind.

Chapter 71

Reiki is Love and Compassion

True compassion is undirected and holds no conceptual focus.
That kind of genuine, true compassion is only possible after
realizing emptiness.
– Tsoknyi Rinpoche, *Carefree Dignity*

The essence of the system of Reiki is love and compassion. We can
see this clearly within the precepts:

Do not anger
Do not worry
Be grateful
Be true to your way and your being
Show compassion to yourself and others

When we soften our anger and worry, we start to slowly become
more compassionate and loving.

And the deepest layer of love and compassion is revealed when
we are loving and compassionate from a non-dualistic state of
mind, a state of mind of emptiness. This is what, as practitioners
and teachers of the system of Reiki, we need to embody more and
more.

But what does love and compassion from a non-dualistic state
of mind mean?

It means simply this: that I am you and you are me. Thus
there is nothing to give – no giver, no receiver and no gift. It also
means that there is no "distance," nothing to bridge, nothing to
send. All of this frees us up from the idea that we need to heal
something; in this space of freedom, we can be completely open
and expanded with no conceptual focus. This in turn allows our

love and compassion to flow more freely, within and without, removing any divisions or barriers our minds may create.

Love and compassion within the system of Reiki is love and compassion without any strings attached to it. Without any idea of an outcome, without labelling, judging, and distinguishing, letting go of these strings sets us free, free to just shine.

The more we teach or learn practices in which we distinguish "ourselves" from "others," the more we see that we are all separate. The more we see this separation, feeling a distance which we need to bridge, the harder it will be to be in a non-dual loving and compassionate state of mind.

True compassion recognizes that all the boundaries we perceive between ourselves and others are an illusion. Compassion is the ability to see the deep connectedness between ourselves and others.

> Moreover, true compassion recognizes that all the boundaries we perceive between ourselves and others are an illusion. When we first begin to practice compassion, this very deep level of understanding may elude us, but we can have faith that if we start where we are, we will eventually feel our way toward it.
> – Madisyn Taylor, *DailyOM: Learning to Live*

This is why the symbols and mantras, the meditations, hands-on healing, the precepts, and the Reiju are all there; they help us to lay bare this non-dual state of love and compassion, so that we have a direct experience of oneness and of being Reiki. And in this state of non-dual love and compassion, we can just shine. When we just shine, there is no need to direct anything, no need to focus on something. We can just be Reiki, be the great bright light of love and compassion.

Chapter 72

How Our Compassionate Mind/heart Affects the World

Find inner peace, and thousands around you will find their salvation.
– St. Seraphim of Sarov

In our modern age we live in such a disconnected state of mind/ heart. We might think we are more interconnected than ever, with Facebook, texting, Instagram and so on. But that is a kind of external connectedness through gadgets. Real connectedness takes place in the mind/heart.

Sometimes our mind/heart is clouded over with feelings of loneliness, separateness, and disconnection. Through practicing meditation we can let go of these clouds and start to rediscover our true mind/heart. Within our true mind/heart, we start to realize that we are all interconnected already.

Mind/heart is described as space in many old spiritual traditions. This means that our true mind/heart is open, without any boundaries, just like space. Our true mind/heart is full of compassion because we have become more open-minded. The more we practice meditation, the more we begin to realize that we are all in the same space. The space I am sitting in right now is the same space you are sitting in. Let's take a closer look at this. I am in my office right now typing away to create this blog. You might say that the space in my office is different than the space in your house. Now let's break down the walls of my office and your house. Now, can we distinguish what was my space and your space? No of course not. Opening our minds is like breaking down the walls that separate us. By investigating the spaciousness of our mind/heart, we realize that we are all interconnected..

Many spiritual traditions also say that: "I am the universe and the universe is me." We can therefore say that our bodies are separate, but our true mind/heart is always interconnected.

Now we come to the juicy bit. If our true mind/heart is always and has always been interconnected, then that also means that whatever I think will affect everything, the entire universe!

In Japanese Tendai Buddhism there is a teaching that says there are three thousand realms in one mind.

> This is the idea that the action of one's mind in a single instant contains "three thousand realms," or the entire universe, and therefore if our mind acts it can affect the entire cosmos.
> – Jiko Kohno, *Right View, Right Life: Insights of a Woman Buddhist Priest*

Therefore if I let go of my anger, worry and fear, if I am more grateful and compassionate, then my mind/heart becomes more calm, loving, and at peace. In turn, everything and everybody can benefit from this. In other words, through something as simple as meditation, we can create harmony and healing in the world.

On the other hand, if my mind/heart is full of anger, worry, and fear, not being grateful and compassionate, then this will create an agitated mind/heart which will have a negative effect on the world.

Through meditation, we can nurture an open spacious mind/heart, where we will not feel lonely, separate, or disconnected. In this way, we can hopefully one day realize internal happiness which, in turn, can heal the world around us.

Glossary of Japanese Terms

Anshin Ritsumei – spiritual peace in our mind/heart, enlightenment

Choku Rei – True Self, direct or straight spirit

Dai Ajari – great esoteric master

Dai Kômyô – great bright light, void, non-duality, emptiness

Darani – mantra, mystic phrase

Deshi – lineage disciple

Gakkai – society

Gassho – putting your palms together, union, non-duality

Gyō – practice, ascetic practices

Hara – stomach, center, true center, center of our True Self

Hatsurei hō – to generate a greater amount of spirit method

Hō – Dharma, method, truth, teachings

Hon sha ze sho nen – I am Right Mind, my original nature is a non-dual thought

Jōshin – focusing the mind

Ki – energy, breath, air, life force

Kokyū – breathing, in and out breath

Ku – emptiness, void

Okuden – hidden or inner teachings

Paramitas, six – the six virtues or perfections of generosity, morality, patience, persistence, concentration, and wisdom

Reiju – spiritual blessing, spiritual offering

Reiki – True Self, spiritual energy

Ryô – to cure, to heal

Sanmitsu – three mysteries of mind, body, and speech/energy

Satori – enlightenment

Sei heki – inclination to remember our True Self

Shinpiden – mystery teachings, not just for teaching but for deepening your personal practice, remembering the mystery of the universe and life

Shoden – beginner's teachings

Tanden – field of elixir, ocean of ki
Toitsu – to unite, to unify
Waka – poetry

Bibliography

Addiss, Stephen. *Zen Sourcebook: Traditional Documents from China, Korea, and Japan*. Indianapolis: Hackett Publishing Company, 2008.

Bowring, Richard. *The Religious Traditions of Japan 500–1600*. Port Melbourne: Cambridge University Press, 2008.

Chowang, Orgyen. *Our Pristine Mind: A Practical Guide to Unconditional Happiness*. Shambhala Publications, Inc., 2016.

Cleary, Thomas. *Zen Essence: The Science of Freedom, Shambhala Dragon Edition*. Boston: Shambhala, 2000.

Davey, HE. *The Teachings of Tempu: Practical Meditation for Daily Life*. Albany: Michi Publishing, 2013.

Deshimaru, Taisen. *Mushotoku Mind: The Heart of the Heart Sutra*. Chino Valley: Hohm Press, 2012.

Doi, Hiroshi. *A Modern Reiki Method for Healing*. Southfield: Vision Publications, 2014.

Gleason, William. *The Spiritual Foundations of Aikido*. Rochester: Destiny Books, 1995.

Goi, Masahisa. *God and Man: Guideposts for Spiritual Peace and Awakening*. Japan: Byakko Press.

Goi, Masahisa. *Living Like the Blue Sky: 5 talks by Masahisa Goi*. Japan: Byakko Press.

Hakeda, Yoshito S. *Kukai: Major Works*. New York: Columbia University Press, 1972.

Hanh, Thich Nhat. *Fear: Essential Wisdom for Getting Through the Storm*. New York: HarperOne, 2012.

Hanh, Thich Nhat. *True Love: A Practice for Awakening the Heart*. Boston: Shambhala Publications, 2004.

Hanh, Thich Nhat. *You Are Here: Discovering the Magic of the Present Moment*. Shambhala Publications, 2010.

Hyers, Conrad. *Once-Born, Twice-Born Zen: The Soto and Rinzai Schools of Japan*. Eugene: WIPF & Stock Publishing, 2004.

Katagiri, Dainin. *Each Moment Is the Universe: Zen and the Way of Being Time*. Boston: Shambhala Publications, 2007.

Katagiri, Dainin. *You Have to Say Something: Manifesting Zen Insight*. Boston: Shambhala Publications, 2000.

Khan, Hazrat Inayat. *The Mysticism of Sound and Music*. Boston: Shambhala Publications, 1996.

Kohno, Jiko. *Right View, Right Life: Insights of a Woman Buddhist Priest*. Tokyo: Kosei Publishing Co., 1998.

Kukai. *Shingon Texts*. Moraga, CA: Numata Center for Buddhist Translation & Research, 2004.

Kwong, Jakusho. *No Beginning, No End: The Intimate Heart of Zen*. Boston: Shambhala Publications, 2003.

Maezumi, Taizan. *Appreciate Your Life: The Essence of Zen Practice*. Boston: Shambhala Publications, 2002.

Maltese, Maurizio. *Zen and the Art of Self Preservation: The Strategies of the Martial Arts*. Milan: Carabá Publishing House, 2014.

Morinaga, Soko. *Novice to Master: An Ongoing Lesson in The Extent of My Own Stupidity*. Somerville: Wisdom Publications, 2002.

Myodo, Satomi. *Passionate Journey: The Spiritual Autobiography of Satomi Myodo*. Boston: Shambhala Publications, 1987.

Oda, Ryuko. *Kaji: Empowerment and Healing in Esoteric Buddhism*. Japan: Kineizan Shinjo-in Mitsumonkai, 1992.

Prasad, Kathleen. *Reiki for Dogs: Using Spiritual Energy to Heal and Vitalize Man's Best Friend*. Berkeley, CA: Ulysses Press, 2012.

Reid, Daniel. *Chi Gung: Harnessing the Power of the Universe*. Boston: Shambhala Publications, 1998.

Shaner, David Edward. *The Bodymind Experience in Japanese Buddhism: A Phenomenological Perspective of Kukai and Dogen*. Albany: State University of New York Press, 1985.

Shinonuma, Ryōjun. *The Life-long Spiritual Journey of an Apprentice Japanese Bonze: Awakening to a new worldview by fulfilling the One-thousand Days Trekking Practice on Mt. Ōmine*. Tokyo: Pro Sophia, 2014.

Smart, Ninian. *World Philosophies*. New York: Routledge, 2008.

Sogyal Rinpoche. *The Tibetan Book of Living and Dying*. New York: HarperCollins, 2009.

Soho, Takuan. *The Unfettered Mind: Writings of the Zen Master to the Sword Master*. Tokyo: Kodansha International, 1986.

Stiene, Bronwen and Frans. *A–Z of Reiki Pocketbook: Everything About Reiki*. Winchester: O-Books, 2006.

Stiene, Bronwen and Frans. *The Japanese Art of Reiki*. Winchester: O-Books, 2005.

Stiene, Bronwen and Frans. *The Reiki Sourcebook*. Winchester: O-Books, 2003.

Stiene, Bronwen and Frans. *Your Reiki Treatment*. Winchester: O-Books, 2007.

Stiene, Frans. *The Inner Heart of Reiki: Rediscovering Your True Self*. Hants: Ayni Books, 2015.

Stone, Jacqueline. *Original Enlightenment and the Transformation of Medieval Japanese Buddhism*. Honolulu: University of Hawaii Press, 2003.

Suzuki, Shunryu. *Not Always So: Practicing the True Spirit of Zen*. New York: HarperCollins, 2002.

Suzuki, Shunryu. *Zen Mind, Beginner's Mind*. New York: Weatherhill, 1970.

Tarthang Tulku. *Openness Mind*. Cazadero: Dharma Publishing, 1990.

Taylor, Madisyn. *DailyOM: Learning to Live*. Carlsbad: Hay House, 2010.

Tohei, Koichi. *Aikido: The Coordination of Mind and Body for Self-defence*. Souvenir Press, 1996.

Tsoknyi Rinpoche. *Carefree Dignity*. Boulder: Rangjung Yeshe Publications, 2013.

Ueshiba, Morihei. *The Art of Peace*. Boston: Shambhala Publications, 2002.

Unno, Taitetsu. *Shin Buddhism: Bits of Rubble Turn into Gold*. Image, 2002.

Wilson, William Scott. *The Demon's Sermon on the Martial Arts*.

Tokyo: Kodansha International, 2006.

Wilson, William Scott. *The Swordsman's Handbook: Samurai Teachings on the Path of the Sword*. Boston: Shambhala Publications, 2014.

Yamakage, Motohisa. *The Essence of Shinto: Japan's Spiritual Heart*. Tokyo: Kodansha International, 2006.

Yamasaki, Taiko. *Shingon: Japanese Esoteric Buddhism*. Boston: Shambhala Publications, 1988.

Yasuo, Yuasa. *The Body, Self-Cultivation, and Ki-Energy*. Albany: State University of New York Press, 1993.

Yen, Sheng. *Attaining the Way: A Guide to the Practice of Chan Buddhism*. Boston: Shambhala Publications, 2006.

Yeshe, Lama Thubten. *When the Chocolate Runs Out*. Somerville: Wisdom Publications, 2011.

Who is Frans Stiene?

Frans has been a major influence on global research into the system of Reiki since the early 2000s. His practical understanding of the Japanese influences on the system has allowed students around the world to connect deeply with this practice.

Students naturally respond to Frans' warmth and intelligence. His own personal spiritual Reiki practice is a model that many students wish to emulate, and offers great encouragement to those on the same path. Frans is a co-founder of the International House of Reiki and Shibumi International Reiki Association with Bronwen Logan (Stiene). He has also co-authored with her the critically acclaimed books *The Reiki Sourcebook*, *The Japanese Art of Reiki*, *A–Z of Reiki Pocketbook*, *Reiki Techniques Card Deck* and *Your Reiki Treatment*.

Originally from Holland, Frans is now mainly based in Australia and since 1998 has trained in a variety of countries such as Japan, Nepal, Italy, UK and Australia. Some of his Reiki teachers include Hyakuten Inamoto, Doi Hiroshi and Chris Marsh. Frans' research has included interviewing Chiyoko Yamaguchi and other Japanese teachers, including Dr. Matsuoka. Although Frans is trained as a Gendai Reiki Ho Shihan (teacher) and a Komyo Reiki Shihan (teacher), he prefers to teach a traditional form of Japanese Reiki, Usui Reiki Ryoho, that he feels reflects a desire to bring the teachings back to their very source, rediscovering our True Self.

Most teachers in Japan teach the system of Reiki from Chujiro Hayashi's viewpoint while Frans tries to teach it as much as possible from Mikao Usui's viewpoint.

Frans is currently training with a Japanese Shingon priest, Takeda Hakusai Ajari, who was once a Tendai monk as a disciple of the great Sakai Dai Ajari, to learn about Shinto, Shugendo, Tendai, and Shingon. Frans is also studying with Reverend Yamabushi Priest Kûban from France.

Frans keeps researching and practicing traditional Japanese teachings to find out what Mikao Usui himself was practicing to get a deeper understanding about what the system of Reiki is really about. This will help him to become a better teacher and to support students in their understanding of the system and their own personal spiritual practice. Frans is one of the rare Reiki teachers who is undertaking these practices.
– Reverend Kûban Jakkôin, Shugendo priest

The contents of what Frans teaches is formed by what has been practiced in Japan since the early 1900s, long before the system of Reiki left Japan, and the researched influences on the system. This particular method includes physical and energy-enhancing exercises to help practitioners delve deeper into their Reiki practice. The earlier teachings consider the system not just to be a hands-on-healing practice but one that also focuses on a student's spiritual path.

The spiritual level of the practitioner directly reflects the effect of Reiki. In a sense, the more you are enlightened, the more the effectiveness of Reiki enhances. The more you practice Reiki for saving others, the brighter your innate light shines to drive away clouds covering your mind. I think this is the quintessence of Reiki. I hope Frans Stiene's way of understanding Reiki spreads in the world to enlighten those who practice Reiki based on a superficial understanding of the tradition.
– Reverend Takeda Hakusai

Frans' open, humorous, and informal style of teaching has been an inspiration for students and clients throughout the USA, Europe, Asia, and Australia. His aim is to provide students with the most comprehensive and up-to-date information about the system of Reiki as well as a strong energetic connection to Mikao Usui's teachings.

Apart from teaching all three levels of the system of Reiki and specialized classes, Frans offers limited one-on-one training sessions for students and one hour hands-on healing sessions all over the word. He also does one-on-one Skype sessions, teaches through teleclasses, and offers retreats. During his retreats you will delve deep into rediscovering your True Self, which is a must if you want to help others. His Shinpiden Reiki III courses are attended by many existing Reiki teachers who want to take their practice to a deeper level.

For more information on all the courses, blogs, etc visit the International House of Reiki website: www.IHReiki.com

Facebook for the International House of Reiki:
www.facebook.com/IHReiki
Facebook of Frans Stiene:
https://www.facebook.com/frans.stiene

What people are saying about

The Inner Heart of Reiki: Rediscovering Your True Self

I am a Tendai monk, the founder of Tendai Sect, Denkyo Daishi Saicho, which stresses Doshin – Heart for the Way – as of most importance. In Denjyutsu Isshin Kaimon, Kojo (Tendai monk, 779–858) quotes Saicho's famous words: "There is livelihood in Doshin, there is Doshin in livelihood." I had the opportunity to spend a week with Frans Stiene upon his visit to Japan, when I had the honor of guiding him through Buddhist practices. I was thoroughly impressed with Frans' Doshin and was struck with awe. In high regards to Frans Stiene's Doshin, I have presented him with the Kesa – monk's stole – which I received upon initiation to priesthood. Kesa is the soul of a priest. Having witnessed his Doshin and soul, both in person and through *The Inner Heart of Reiki: Rediscovering Your True Self*, I look forward to Frans' further endeavors. Reiki is not merely a "technique," but has a vital role in guiding one to reach "perfection as a human being." The idea contained in the precepts, "Just for today, do not anger, do not worry…" also is reflected in One Day, One Life by my teacher, Sakai Yusai Dai Ajari. If you want to know whether a teacher is a true Reiki teacher or not, all you have to do is to ask him what the True Self is. Without the trustworthy insight of the True Self, nobody can insist he or she is a true disciple of Mikao Usui. This book testifies that the author is one of the true Reiki teachers.
Takeda Hakusai Ajari

The Inner Heart of Reiki resonated deeply within me, for I have always believed that we are all one and that Oneness is the essence of our universe. In this book Frans Stiene takes us on a journey through Japanese Buddhist teachings and meanings of mantras and kanji as taught by Mikao Usui. It is a journey back to our True Self, Oneness and being Reiki rather than living in duality and just doing Reiki. This book is a must-read not just for Reiki Practitioners and Teachers but for everyone who is on life's journey of discovery. So much of Frans' research, study, and practice are openly shared with the reader. Frans does not just talk the talk; he genuinely walks the walk.

The Australian Reiki Connection Inc. is pleased to endorse *The Inner Heart of Reiki* to its members and to the Reiki community.

John Coleman, president of Australian Reiki Connection Inc., Australia's leading Reiki association.

Every once in a while you find a book that changes everything. It is almost like you have a paradigm shift, and you take the words into your new understanding of how the world could be. Things that you always questioned come clearer even though you did not know that there was confusion. Frans Stiene's new book *The Inner Heart of Reiki* is just such a book. Every page took me deeper into myself and lit up the places where there were shadows of doubt about the system of Reiki and the spiritual path that I am on.

I have studied Buddhism for a number of years and have been working on becoming a Zen priest for the past few years. I also have a yoga studio and have trained in yoga for the past 20 years. Neither Zen nor yoga have been able to take me as close to my true nature as Reiki has done. When asked what religion I am, I say I am a Reiki Buddhist for that reason.

In Buddhism there is a well-renowned sutra called the Diamond Sutra. It is called the Diamond Sutra because it cuts through delusion. This book is similar in that it cuts through the delusion and hype of typical Reiki books and goes right to the core of what Reiki really is, a spiritual path. This book hits the mark and the mark, it turns out, is the true self. Frans has gone further than anyone in the world to study and learn about the system of Reiki and it shows on every page, always bringing us back to our True Self, inviting readers to explore for themselves what the true essence is all about. We are fortunate that Frans has done the research for us and we can all follow the path that he has cleared for us. I have decided that I will not teach anyone the third level of Reiki unless they have read this book, because if they have not we cannot have a good conversation of what the deeper elements of the system of Reiki are, so there would be no reason to advance anyone to that level.

Jeff Emerson, Reiki and yoga teacher, author of *Unfolding the Lotus*

This is a must-read for all students of the system of Reiki. Frans, through his research and practice, has peeled away the myths about the system of Reiki and gives us a clear understanding of the Reiki journey. He also shows how meditation practice is a fundamental part of the system. This book is just what the Reiki world needs, written by someone who walks his talk.

Helen Galpin, co-founder of the British School of Meditation

Having investigated The Great Way of the Asians in shamanism, Daoism, Buddhism, medicine, ancient science, Tai Chi and Qigong since 1963–4, I have a special appreciation of any "system" that articulates the natural presence of the truth and power of the Universe within a context of Self. Versions of self-discovery, self-awareness, ultimate personal potential and the revelation of the True Self – from Lao Zi and Daoists, to Shakyamuni and the Buddhist flourishing, to the great Zen monks and poets – all point to the same views, insights and practices. Mikao Usui's Way is one of those beautiful articulations of the mastery of the nature of human experience and the True Self. Frans Stiene has done us a huge favor by revealing the actual context of Reiki as a Way of Self-Cultivation which is primarily focused on refinement of self which happens to include a method of helping and healing others that is a secondary feature of The Way.

Dr. Roger Jahnke, OMD, founder/director of the Institute of

Integral Qigong and Tai Chi (IIQTC); author of *The Healer Within* and *The Healing Promise of Qi*; http:/IIQTC.org

Frans Stiene is an inspiring teacher because he embodies the spiritual gift of Reiki in all his actions and throughout his day, not just when giving someone a session. In this delightful book he weaves the threads of the rich history of Japanese spiritual practices that have brought him to this inner sacred space.
Neil McKinney, MD, author of *Naturopathic Oncology*

Frans Stiene is one of the world's premier Reiki teachers and this book is a window into one of his amazing classes. One of Frans' special gifts is to make extremely profound spiritual truths easily accessible. This book will awaken readers to the deeper possibilities of their Reiki practice and offer techniques to help them get there. A must-read for anyone interested in Reiki practice!
Kathleen Prasad, founder of Animal Reiki Source, president of Shelter Animal Reiki Association

The Inner Heart of Reiki is a wonderful companion for the advanced Reiki student and/or teacher who wants to dive deeper into their daily practice and expand their energetic understanding of Reiki. This book is a clear and concise guide to help you integrate the various components of the system of Reiki – the precepts, meditations, symbols/mantras, and hands-on-healing – into your sessions, classes, and most importantly, your life. Frans Stiene, often referred to as "the Reiki Teacher's Teacher," takes his extensive research and grounded personal understanding and practice, and outlines a path of practice you can follow in his gentle, compassionate, and often humorous way. As a Reiki teacher and practitioner, I found this book quite breathtaking. Breathtaking is the perfect word – this book reminds you to connect to your breath and your True Self while reading it! The book was truly wonderful, and something I'll reread and refer to often as I expand my personal understanding of Reiki.

Deborah Flanagan, Reiki teacher and author of *Building a Powerful Practice: Successful Strategies for Your Wellness Business*

Frans Stiene illuminates the intricacies of Reiki with the insight and simple elegance of a master. His writing resonates with the depth of experience.

Barry Lancet, award-winning author of *Japantown*

AYNI BOOKS

AYNI BOOKS
ALTERNATIVE HEALTH & HEALING

"Ayni" is a Quechua word meaning "reciprocity" - sharing, giving and receiving - whatever you give out comes back to you. To be in Ayni is to be in balance, harmony and right relationship with oneself and nature, of which we are all an intrinsic part. Complementary and Alternative approaches to health and well-being essentially follow a holistic model, within which one is given support and encouragement to move towards a state of balance, true health and wholeness, ultimately leading to the awareness of one's unique place in the Universal jigsaw of life - Ayni, in fact. If you have enjoyed this book, why not tell other readers by posting a review on your preferred book site. Recent bestsellers from AYNI Books are:

Reclaiming Yourself from Binge Eating
A Step-By-Step Guide to Healing
Leora Fulvio, MFT
Win the war against binge eating, wake up each morning at peace with your body, unafraid of food and overeating.
Paperback: 978-1-78099-680-6 ebook: 978-1-78099-681-3

The Reiki Sourcebook (revised ed.)
Frans Stiene, Bronwen Stiene
A popular, comprehensive and updated manual for the Reiki novice, teacher and general reader.
Paperback: 978-1-84694-181-8 ebook: 978-1-84694-648-6

The Chakras Made Easy
Hilary H. Carter

From the successful Made Easy series, *Chakras Made Easy* is a practical guide to healing the seven chakras.

Paperback: 978-1-78099-515-1 ebook: 978-1-78099-516-8

The Inner Heart of Reiki
Rediscovering Your True Self

Frans Stiene

A unique journey into the inner heart of the system of Reiki, to help practitioners and teachers rediscover their True Selves.

Paperback: 978-1-78535-055-9 ebook: 978-1-78535-056-6

Middle Age Beauty
Soulful Secrets from a Former Face Model Living Botox Free in Her Forties

Machel Shull

Find out how to look fabulous during middle age without plastic surgery by learning inside secrets from a former model.

Paperback: 978-1-78099-574-8 ebook: 978-1-78099-575-5

The Optimized Woman
Using Your Menstrual Cycle to Achieve Success and Fulfillment

Miranda Gray

If you want to get ahead, get a cycle! For women who want to create life-success in a female way.

Paperback: 978-1-84694-198-6

The Patient in Room Nine Says He's God
Louis Profeta

A roller coaster ride of joy, controversy, triumph and tragedy; often all on the same page.

Paperback: 978-1-84694-354-6 ebook: 978-1-78099-736-0

Re-humanizing Medicine
A Holistic Framework for Transforming Your Self, Your Practice,
and the Culture of Medicine
David Raymond Kopacz
Re-humanizing medical practice for doctors, clinicians, clients, and
systems.
Paperback: 978-1-78279-075-4 ebook: 978-1-78279-074-7

You Can Beat Lung Cancer Using Alternative/Integrative Interventions
Carl O. Helvie R.N., Dr.P.H.
Significantly increase your chances of long-term lung cancer survival by using holistic alternative and integrative interventions by
physicians or health practitioners.
Paperback: 978-1-78099-283-9 ebook: 978-1-78099-284-6

Readers of ebooks can buy or view any of these bestsellers by
clicking on the live link in the title. Most titles are published in
paperback and as an ebook. Paperbacks are available in traditional
bookshops. Both print and ebook formats are available online.

Find more titles and sign up to our readers' newsletter at
http://www.johnhuntpublishing.com/mind-body-spirit
Follow us on Facebook at https://www.facebook.com/OBooks
and Twitter at https://twitter.com/obooks